Yoga Teaching Handbook

of related interest

Yoga for a Happy Back
A Teacher's Guide to Spinal Health through Yoga Therapy
Rachel Krentzman, PT, E-RYT
Foreword by Aadil Palkhivala
ISBN 978 1 84819 271 3
eISBN 978 0 85701 253 1

The Supreme Art and Science of Raja and Kriya Yoga
The Ultimate Path to Self-Realisation
Stephen Sturgess
Foreword by Dr David Frawley
ISBN 978 1 84819 261 4
eISBN 978 0 85701 209 8

Mudras of Yoga
72 Hand Gestures for Healing and Spiritual Growth
Cain Carroll with Revital Carroll
ISBN 978 1 84819 176 1 (card set)
eISBN 978 0 85701 143 5

Yoga Teaching Handbook

A Practical Guide for Yoga Teachers and Trainees

Edited by Sian O'Neill

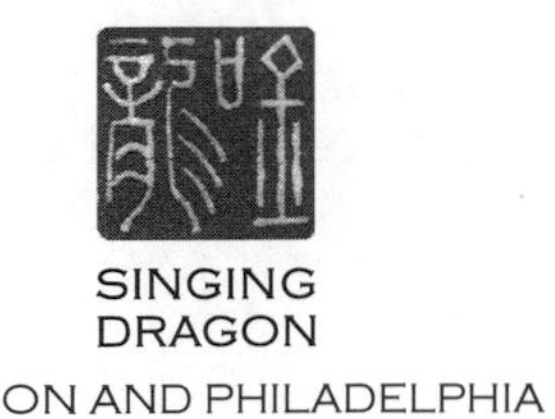

SINGING DRAGON
LONDON AND PHILADELPHIA

Disclaimer: Every effort has been made to ensure that the information contained in this book is correct, but it should not in any way be substituted for medical advice. Readers should always consult a qualified medical practitioner before adopting any physical therapies. Neither the author nor the publisher takes responsibility for any consequences of any decision made as a result of the information contained in this book.

First published in 2018
by Singing Dragon
an imprint of Jessica Kingsley Publishers
73 Collier Street
London N1 9BE, UK
and
400 Market Street, Suite 400
Philadelphia, PA 19106, USA

www.singingdragon.com

Library of Congress Cataloging in Publication Data
Names: O'Neill, Sian, editor.
Title: Yoga teaching handbook : a practical guide for yoga teachers and trainees / edited by Sian O'Neill.
Description: London ; Philadelphia : Singing Dragon, [2018] | Includes bibliographical references and index.
Identifiers: LCCN 2017022816 | ISBN 9781848193550 (alk. paper)
Subjects: LCSH: Hatha yoga--Study and teaching.
Classification: LCC RA781.7 .Y634 2018 | DDC 613.7/046076--
dc23 LC record available at https://lccn.loc.gov/2017022816

British Library Cataloguing in Publication Data
A CIP catalogue record for this book is available from the British Library

ISBN 978 1 84819 355 0
eISBN 978 0 85701 313 2

Printed and bound in the United States

Contents

Introduction

Sian O'Neill

The idea for this book came when I was sitting in a café with a blank piece of paper, a coffee and a pen. I was experimenting with disconnecting from the internet and social media; phone to one side. I realised that what I would find really useful is a practical book on teaching yoga including tips and lessons learned from experienced teachers. Yoga teachers generally like yoga books. There are not many texts, however, on the practicalities of running your yoga business, large or small. This book is an attempt to meet that need. We have been fortunate enough to assemble a panel of some of the world's best-known and loved teachers. Every one of our contributors is a highly experienced yoga teacher and I am so grateful to them for sharing their knowledge and experience.

Yoga is more popular than ever with many also choosing the path of teaching yoga. It is a privilege to teach yoga, but as anyone who is already teaching or contemplating teaching yoga knows, it also comes with its own set of challenges and responsibilities. How do you come up with new and creative sequences each week? How do you safely incorporate students with injuries without overstepping boundaries? And for those of you thinking of expanding your yoga business to run retreats, how do you plan a safe and enjoyable retreat, from which students return refreshed, without burning out yourself? Our contributors address these and many other issues – I hope you take away some practical gems.

I write this having recently returned from the British Wheel of Yoga Annual Congress, the theme for which this year was 'transformation'. The congress caused me to reflect on how yoga has changed me – from that first blissful feeling in *Savasana* to the recognition that yoga has changed both me and my relationship with the world. It is this, I think, that is so powerful about teaching yoga: the potential to affect people's lives so positively. Perhaps it is the under-confident student who is helped through yoga, someone going through a period of intense change or the student managing to carve out that precious hour or so of yoga amidst a super-hectic schedule. We know that everyone who turns up in class has prioritised yoga over all the other possible options in a commitment to their wellbeing. Yoga offers this amazing toolkit to help us and our students through the vagaries of life with all of its ups and downs.

Rather than attempting to summarise the chapters that follow, I shall let the contributions speak for themselves. If there is one theme, though, that is repeated in different chapters and in conversations with contributing teachers, it is around intention and knowing why you are teaching yoga. What is it that has led you to want to teach? And what is it that you want to offer students? Each of us will have a different answer to these questions, which will inform how we shape our yoga teaching path.

I know that I have learned a great deal in putting this book together. I hope you also find something similarly useful inside to support your own yoga teaching career. Happy reading!

I would like to thank all of our contributors for their time, commitment and thoughtful chapters. Special thanks are also owed to Sarah Hamlin at Jessica Kingsley Publishers for her professionalism, support and thoughtful input, to Victoria Peters and Sophie Raoufi, and also to Jessica Kingsley herself for believing in and supporting the idea from the start. Last and not least, thank you to Alex.

Please do get in touch with any comments or feedback – I would love to hear from you (you can reach me on sianoneill@yahoo.co.uk).

A note on transliteration

In transliterating Sanskrit words into Western script, we have followed the convention of the International Alphabet of Sanskrit Transliteration (IAST) (except for words – such as 'vinyasa' – that have found their way into the Oxford English Dictionary, where we have used the common English form without diacritical markings). There are numerous guides to the correct pronunciation of transliterated Sanskrit words available online. Sanskrit nouns have been rendered in their base form without declension, irrespective of their function in the sentence. Accordingly, although the plural of Sanskrit nouns is not technically formed with the suffix '*-s*', we have followed the widespread practice in English language texts of showing plurals by the addition of '*-s*', to the base form of the noun.

— 1 —

Influence and Evolution

Lizzie Lasater

The ethics of teaching yoga amidst the shifting mediums of our profession.

In the last hundred years, the profession of *yoga teacher* has undergone substantial transnational and cultural transformations. In this relatively short span of time, I can trace my lineage and my influence from one-on-one mentorship in India with Krishnamacharya, to co-ed group classes with BKS Iyengar, to mixed-style commercial studios like YogaWorks in Los Angeles, to digital learning platforms like YogaGlo.

To borrow conceptually from the modernist philosopher, Marshall McLuhan, this transformation indicates a shift in the *medium* of transmission.[1] Doesn't it therefore follow that the *message* itself has also changed? In other words, as we teach yoga differently, does *what* we teach also change? When I think about practicing and teaching yoga as a woman in the West, conflicts and questions arise about authenticity, ownership, orientalism, and ethics.

If we acknowledge that an evolution in both medium and message is underway, my question becomes: what does it mean to be a professional yoga teacher today? How can we best support our students to find silence in the midst of our cacophonous 21st century? How do we make space for the unseen inner work of yoga in a culture ever more mesmerized by materiality and consumerism? And how can we personally integrate a profession about slowing down into our accelerating lives?

In short, how can we honor the wisdom of the past while unabashedly living in the evolving present? An alternative title of this chapter might have been: 'Can we teach *samādhi* on social media?'

My answer is to create an intention. I hope that our professional conduct can, in and of itself, facilitate a deepening of our personal yoga practice. The dream is to establish a dynamic of integration so that it becomes possible for our work to feed our practice and our practice to feed our work, thus ultimately enhancing our lives.

What follows is my personal manifesto: eight points on the ethics of teaching amidst the shifting mediums of our profession.

At the end of each class, my mom, Judith Hanson Lasater, says, 'May we live like the lotus, at home in the muddy water.' I've adopted this saying when I teach as well – partially as an homage to my lineage, but also because I like its honesty. I like the open acknowledgement that our life and our practice are muddy, but this bittersweetness is precisely what makes them rich.

My practice is at the heart of my teaching

When we moved into our current apartment, it was partially furnished with many attractive, mid-century modern pieces. My architect husband wanted to keep them all. But I insisted on moving half of the furniture out to make space for yoga. That's exactly what I kept saying: 'I need empty space to practice yoga.'

This physical space is a symbol for the mental, emotional, and psychological space that yoga practice both requires and creates. I sometimes think of my home practice as a controlled environment to experience emptiness. It is a way that I have found to step into the unknown each day – by creating a fence around an open field.

My practice is a unique time in my day when I don't need to accomplish or produce anything. I'm not busy distracting myself by texting or talking or eating or cleaning. Instead, I can drop all of the roles I usually play: wife, daughter, sister, friend, business partner, colleague, neighbour, citizen. For these few minutes, I don't need to be anything to anybody. I am simply in relationship with my Self.

In this way, my mat is a private laboratory for experimentation. Donna Farhi summarises this idea by saying: 'Yoga is a pragmatic science where everything is tested and verified through direct experience.'[2] It is precisely this *direct experience* that I want to inform my teaching. In my view, teaching yoga is 80 percent practice and 20 percent technique.

To teach from your own experience takes courage. It's a form of honesty to offer your students an idea or movement or sequence that you didn't receive from your teachers but instead developed in the laboratory of your own practice. But that's where it gets interesting. That's where it becomes juicy and wild and unknown. That's exactly where I want to live.

Becoming a mirror

We have the great fortune of teaching a subject that can have a profound impact on our students' lives. Encountering this ourselves is often what drew us more deeply into yoga in the first place. But it's important to remember that the yoga itself is the magic, not me as the teacher.

When I go home after teaching a workshop I sometimes receive emails from students expressing gratitude. They can contain touching accounts of a healing shift that the student experienced in my class. While these notes can be flattering, they are also tricky because they often give *me* credit for creating the positive experience.

Mom likes to say that the primary job of a yoga teacher is to 'mirror back the inherent wisdom and inner goodness of each student'.[3] I like this image because it reminds me that I am not creating anything. Instead, my job is to help my students to find what is already there.

The image of a mirror also implies that on some level, my work is to disappear. This isn't meant to be self-effacing. But if I want my students to become independent, to be able to build their own self-sustaining practice, then I must help them to see that the deep inner work of yoga has very little to do with the teacher. I want them to see that they themselves are capable of creating the healing magic of yoga.

The more I learn, the more I can teach

I sometimes think of myself as a professional yoga student. After all, when I attend a workshop or take a class or roll out my mat at home, I'm also working to become a better teacher. I like to remind myself that the more deeply I dive into my own practice, the more I have to offer my students. The more I learn, the more I can teach.

I was 22 years old when I completed a 200-hour yoga teacher training program and began teaching classes at YogaWorks in Los Angeles. When I think back to those early years, I sometimes cringe. My style was earnest but so inexperienced. But what I lacked in originality, I made up for in strenuousness. Once, after telling my mom about a sequence I'd just taught, she said with a laugh: 'Well, at least your students are young; you probably didn't kill them.'

This story illustrates a little discussed dynamic in our field. Completing a 200-hour teacher training program does not *make* you a yoga teacher. It is little more than an invitation to *begin to learn* how to teach yoga. It is an early step in a lifelong journey.

Cultivating curiosity and humility are core values that can enrich my teaching and my life. They help me remember to continually see myself as a *student* of yoga, no matter how many years I teach. I actively look for learning opportunities off the yoga mat that put me in touch with the sensations of being a raw beginner. In recent years I've focused on learning German and how to ski, for example. These experiences help me grow empathy for my beginning students.

Function follows form

Injuries are a dark side of our profession. I feel ashamed every time I hear another story of a student who has been hurt during a yoga class. In my analysis, the damage is often caused by misguided alignment instructions or inappropriately forceful adjustments. As I discuss my perspective about touching students in the following section of this chapter, I will focus my attention here on the importance of understanding alignment.

When I talk about correct alignment, I don't mean *correct* based on the specific ideas of one school of yoga over the other. Instead, my emphasis is to look at the anatomy and physiology of the human body. The structures themselves have so much to tell us about the function of joints and muscle groups. In this case, function always follows form.

It is paramount that we as teachers remain willing to respectfully test and question the alignment instructions that we have received. So many of us offer instructions simply because that's what we learned from our teachers. What if we applied this logic to the medical profession? What if an older doctor told you she didn't want to use contemporary chemotherapy methods because that wasn't what she learned from her mentor in the 1980s? This sounds completely nonsensical, right? Well that's exactly what we're doing when we teach *āsana* based solely on inherited instructions.

I want to inform my *āsana* with a deep understanding of functional movement in the human body. This focus breaks the cycle of believing unwaveringly in received alignment ideas. My project, as I begin to train other teachers, is to place more emphasis on learning anatomy and physiology. My intention for myself and my students is to develop movement literacy. I hope you'll join me.

'No' is a complete sentence

Before I touch a student in my yoga class, I ask permission. I actually say these words out loud: 'May I touch you?' You might think it sounds dorky. I certainly did in the beginning. Because this practice deviates from the cultural norm of so many yoga classes, it took me a long time to integrate it into my teaching. But allow me to illustrate the importance of asking permission to touch by enumerating why I think it's a valuable habit and then to examine the function of touch itself in a yoga class.

First, asking permission to touch is good for me as the teacher. It slows me down when I interact with students. And it encourages me to be more conscious with my hands. Second, it reminds the students of their own participation and responsibility in the learning dance. Third, I hope it begins to allow a space for students to say 'no'. This simple word empowers the student to take care of herself by advocating for the boundaries she needs. Lastly, I like asking permission to touch because it signals to everyone else in the class that I will also honor their autonomy.

The most common way I use touch is to give the student information. After asking permission, I will gently touch a student's back kidneys, for example, and suggest that she might enjoy softening *here*. This type of touch is simply to help the student locate her kidneys in three-dimensional space.

The second category of touch that I use is to provide direction. I might, in a seated twist for example, lightly touch someone's left shoulder blade with my hand and say 'move away from my hand' to deepen the twist. In this case I'm not exerting any force and the entire movement comes from the student herself.

The third type of touch is adjustments. This is when I use my strength as an external force to move the student more deeply into a pose. This is the most potentially injurious form of touch and I therefore almost never use this type of touch. Weighed against the potential risks, I have to wonder, what exactly is to be gained? If the student goes more deeply into a backbend, for example, perhaps achieving a so-called 'final pose', whose victory is it really?

Be careful what you say

Teaching yoga is mostly about talking. Of course we demonstrate and gesticulate and touch with our bodies as well, but the primary activity of our job is speaking. As a new teacher, I was so focused on *what* I was saying – worried about sequencing and cuing – that I generally ignored the *quality* of my words.

Reassured by repetitions, I now trust that when I open my mouth in a yoga class, something will come out. My focus has therefore shifted to selecting the type of words and images I want to employ when I teach. It's quite different to ask our students to 'bend' or to 'surrender' forward into *Paschimottanasana*, for example. Or in a standing pose, we can encourage students to 'cut' their outer foot into the floor in *Vīrabhadrāsana II*, but I prefer a less violent word variation like 'anchor'.

Another priority when I teach is to choose words that are about inspiration rather than coercion. In offering a more challenging variation of a pose that might only be appropriate for some students, I'm highly sensitive to the words I use to frame this choice. I never want my students to take an inappropriate variation because they felt pushed. That's simply not a dynamic I want to indulge.

In essence, selecting the colour and tone of the words I use when I teach has become a playful practice. This awareness game draws me more deeply into the present when I'm teaching, which has secondary effects that I like very much.

Love and light won't pay the rent

Teaching yoga is a joy. It's deliciously stimulating and rewarding. It can even be a calling. We often feel that we receive more from our students than we give. But it's also a job. And the yoga industry is a business.

Because yoga sits partially in the spiritual world and trades in images of *love and light*, teachers often receive signals and pressure that we should not be interested in money. The problem is that we can't use *love and light* to pay the rent or our self-employed healthcare premiums or for organic avocado toast.

My highest value in doing business is clarity. I aim to be as straightforward as possible with my expectations and invite my business partners to do the same. When I feel discomfort arise around discussing money, I take notice. This muddy place has potential for growth. I don't want to run away from the world but instead to learn to blossom right here in the midst of the marketplace.

You cannot practice yoga without a body

When I tell a new acquaintance that I teach yoga, I often notice their eye contact waiver as they shift focus to glance at my body. This split-second appraisal is deeply uncomfortable. I'm left imagining their assessment of my figure and projecting all of my insecurities onto this interaction. Does the way I look match up with their preconceptions about what a yoga teacher *should* look like? In other words, do they think that I look thin enough to teach yoga?

For years I resisted committing myself to earning my living from teaching yoga because I was afraid of building a career so focused on my body. I thought this would augment my tendencies towards incessant attention on healthy eating and my weight. I was worried that teaching yoga would drain the pleasure out of my life. And I was convinced that this career choice would ensure eating dinner and drinking a glass of wine would become a battleground of good and evil.

Creating a kinder relationship with my body is an unfolding process. The intention is to become soft and invite a quality of playfulness and appreciation. Dear thighs, thank you for carrying me to the top of mountains. To that end, this Geneen Roth quote helps summarize my focus: 'You are not a mistake. You are not a problem to be solved. But you won't discover this until you are willing to stop banging your head against the wall of shaming and caging and fearing yourself.'[4]

The simple paradox is that yoga is a corporeal practice that is both *about* and *not about* the body. You cannot practice yoga without a body. And as teachers, we are not a separate species from our students. The more we see and embrace our own flaws, the more compassion we will have for those of our students.

The work is to cultivate more kindness towards our own physical incarnation and to share that gentleness with our students. The work is to take meditation and silence more seriously, learning to slow down within our accelerating culture. And the work is to remain deeply curious, offering open hearts and soft eyes to our students. It's wonderful work; I'm so grateful to share this profession with you.

Sending you a deep namaste,
Lizzie
Salzburg, Austria
April 2017

Notes

1 McLuhan, M. (1964) *Understanding Media: The Extensions of Man.* New York: Mentor.

2 Farhi, D. (2006) *Teaching Yoga: Exploring the Teacher–Student Relationship.* Berkeley, CA: Rodmell Press. p.10.

3 Personal communication with Judith Hanson Lasater, Ph.D., PT.

4 Roth, G. (2011) *Women, Food and God: An Unexpected Path to Almost Everything.* New York: Scribner. p.84.

— 2 —

Breath

Andrew McGonigle

The respiratory system

The respiratory system lies within the thorax and is made up of a collection of airways, lung tissue, musculature and blood vessels that allow gas exchange to take place between the air in our environment and our blood. Oxygen is supplied to our tissues to allow our cells to release energy from the food that we ingest and carbon dioxide is released into the environment as a waste product. By regulating the levels of carbon dioxide in the blood, we also regulate the pH or acid-base balance of our body. This is an essential part of homeostasis that involves maintaining a narrow parameter of environmental factors to allow our bodily systems to function optimally.

The respiratory system is the only system in our body to have both voluntary and involuntary control. When we are asleep, or awake but not conscious of our breathing, it is still occurring in the background without our control. But we can also manipulate the breath, particularly during our *āsana* or *prāṇāyāma* practice. We can lengthen, shorten or retain the inhalation or the exhalation. We cannot directly slow our heart rate or speed up our digestion through conscious control, but we can access these systems via the breath. We'll look at how this works in some detail later in the chapter.

As yoga practitioners who recognise the great importance of breathing on and off the mat, we can easily forget that most of the human population may spend their entire lives rarely taking a conscious breath. When we are not conscious of our breath, it is often shallow, only involving the uppermost parts of our chest cavity. This is commonly known as 'chest breathing'. The process of gas exchange here is inefficient since we are only using a small amount of the complete surface area of our lungs, and the lung tissue here has a lesser blood supply than parts of the lungs closer to the base of the chest cavity. The less efficient the gas exchange, the more rapidly we need to breathe and therefore the quicker our heart needs to beat. This not only impacts the heart itself but, since heart rate is synonymous with blood pressure, our blood pressure also rises as a result. Our breath is also very closely linked to our emotions. When we are anxious we tend to adopt shallow chest breathing, but when we do this we can often feel anxious as a result. Thankfully, the reverse of this is also true: as we slow our breathing we tend to feel calmer and more restored.

As a yoga teacher, one of my main goals is to create a space where my students can observe, connect to and enhance their breath. I see yoga as primarily a breathing practice and my teaching revolves around this theme. Yoga is often viewed through the media as being all about flexibility or perfecting a challenging arm balance. Having flexibility is wonderful and arm balances are fun and can help to develop confidence, control and stamina, but without a focus on the breath the practice becomes more like a form of gymnastics. Approaching yoga as a breath-led practice where the movements follow the breath and not the other way around can be a powerful tool to allow students to develop deeper awareness of this vital function.

The anatomy of our airways

Breathing is a mechanical process by which air is drawn in and out of the lungs, while respiration is a chemical process that occurs at a cellular level. To look at breathing in more detail we need to start by reviewing the anatomy of our airways and lungs.

The journey begins at our nostrils. Our nasal cavities have a large surface area full of blood capillaries, cilia, mucus and turbinates that help to warm, filter and moisten the air and direct the flow to the back of the throat. When inhaling through the mouth, it can feel as if you are taking in a larger volume of air but it is more difficult for this air to reach deeper parts of your lungs. When exhaling through the mouth, we tend to lose moisture and heat alongside the exhaled air. Once the inhaled air reaches the back of the throat it has two options: to pass into the larynx at the top of the trachea or windpipe or pass down the oesophagus or food pipe. The epiglottis makes this decision for us and covers the oesophagus that leads to the stomach so that the air can pass down towards the trachea. Similarly, when we are swallowing, the epiglottis covers the larynx so that saliva, food or drink doesn't pass in this direction. Once air reaches the larynx it passes through the glottis, in which the vocal cords are found. A gentle constriction of this area increases the speed of the air passing through and encourages the air to travel deeper into the lungs as a result. The trachea or windpipe is ringed with cartilage that prevents it from collapsing under the air pressure and at its base it splits into two main bronchi, one travelling towards each lung. The bronchi divide further into bronchioles like branches of a tree and eventually we reach the alveoli or air sacs. A pair of lungs can contain up to 700 million of these alveoli, with a surface area the size of a tennis court.

The mechanics of breathing

Our lungs are passive tissue that does not contain muscle and they are separated from the chest wall by a pleural cavity that has a lower pressure than the pressure inside the lungs. This pressure difference creates a vacuum between the lungs and the chest cavity and forces the lungs to track the movement of the chest cavity.

The diaphragm lies in a dome-like shape underneath the lungs and separates the chest cavity from the abdominal cavity. It is the primary muscle of inspiration. As the diaphragm contracts it subtly flattens and at the same time the external intercostal muscles that lie between the ribs tilt the ribs upwards and apart. These movements result in the chest cavity volume increasing and therefore the lungs expand as a result. As the volume of the lungs increases, the pressure inside the lungs decreases. The air pressure in the environment outside the body is now higher than the pressure inside the lungs and air will always move from an area of high to low pressure. Air is therefore drawn into the lungs and we call this inhalation.

Our natural exhalation is passive, involving relaxation of both the external intercostal muscles and the diaphragm. As the chest cavity volume decreases, the lung volume decreases, resulting in the pressure inside the lungs increasing. Air now moves from high to low pressure and exits the lungs into the environment.

In yoga we add to this by making the exhalation active. This involves the action of the internal intercostal muscles that draw the ribs down towards each other and the pelvic floor and deep core muscles that increase the pressure inside the abdominal cavity, assisting the diaphragm to go back to its resting shape more quickly and forcibly. The active exhale expires a greater volume of air from the lungs, allowing for a greater volume to then be inhaled again. This makes the process of gas exchange more efficient and helps to recycle the residual volume of air that must remain in the lungs to prevent the walls from sticking to each other.

Types of breathing and their impact on our nervous system

We touched on the potential emotional effects of predominantly breathing into the upper parts of our chest earlier in the chapter, but let's now look at how this type of breathing can impact our nervous system. Chest breathing stimulates a part of our nervous system known as the sympathetic nervous system, often referred to as our 'fight or flight' response. The sympathetic nervous system increases our heart rate and respiratory rate and sends blood to our muscles so that we can prepare to fight or take flight! Any system that is not essential in that moment, i.e. the digestive, immune and reproductive systems, essentially get shut down. This is one of the reasons why it is so common for people with chronic stress to develop problems with their digestion, immunity and reproductive health. The good news is that there is an opposing system called the parasympathetic nervous system or 'rest and digest' response that balances out the effects of the sympathetic nervous system. The parasympathetic nervous system decreases our heart rate and respiratory rate and stimulates our digestive, immune and reproductive systems. In order to stimulate the parasympathetic nervous system via our respiratory system, we need to adopt either 'belly' or 'diaphragmatic' breathing.

As the diaphragm contracts and flattens, it not only impacts the chest cavity but also increases the pressure inside the abdominal cavity below. When the abdominal muscles are relaxed, the abdomen will respond by expanding its anterior wall forward and out. As the diaphragm relaxes and domes, the pressure exerted on the abdominal cavity decreases and the anterior wall falls back to its original position. This is commonly known as 'belly breathing'. Its advantages over chest breathing are that it encourages more air to reach the lower bases of the lungs, which have a richer blood supply, and therefore gas exchange becomes more efficient. The pressure exerted on the abdominal cavity also stimulates the vagus nerve as it travels through the abdomen. The vagus nerve is the main parasympathetic nerve in the body and helps us to calm and restore the effects of the sympathetic nervous system. Belly breathing is wonderful to adopt when we are practising *āsana* that do not require the active support of our core muscles, such as Savasana or any restorative yoga *āsana*.

We can take this a step further by keeping a gentle contraction of the abdominal muscles as we inhale. The diaphragm is now unable to flatten directly down but instead pushes the lower ribcage out laterally and posteriorly. Acting almost like bellows this expansion of the ribcage is known as 'diaphragmatic breathing'. Air is drawn even deeper into the lower and posterior parts of the lungs and added pressure to the abdominal cavity further improves what is known as 'vagal tone', i.e. the efficiency of the vagus nerve. Diaphragmatic breathing is effective during more active *āsana* practice where we rely on the support of our core musculature.

When we inhale, our heart rate increases via the sympathetic nervous system and when we exhale, our heart rate decreases via the parasympathetic nervous system. This is known as Respiratory Sinus Arrhythmia. In yoga we use this to our advantage by lengthening the exhalation to at least match the length of the inhalation. Many *prāṇāyāma* practices involve lengthening the exhalation so it is longer than the inhalation, further increasing the effects of the parasympathetic nervous system.

Using our breath as a focal point during our *āsana* or meditation practice can help to take our mind off perceived stressful thoughts that trigger the sympathetic nervous system, allowing the calming effects of the parasympathetic nervous system to take effect.

How to incorporate breath into an *āsana* practice

There are many different and effective approaches to introducing breath into a breath-led practice. The suggestions below are based on my own teaching experience over the last decade and I hope they will serve as a helpful foundation when you are exploring your own methods.

A good starting point is to simply encourage your students to begin to observe their natural breath without changing it. This can take place while the students are in a comfortable supine or seated position or standing in *Tāḍāsana*, Mountain Pose. Closing the eyes can really help here, but remember that this doesn't always feel comfortable for everyone so give it as an option. It can be interesting to explore the quality, length and depth of the breath and notice the parts of the body that naturally move with the inhalation and exhalation. Is the breath focused on a particular area of the rib cage? Does the breathing rate fluctuate? One of the aims of the observation is to help the student to develop awareness of their default breathing patterns during both the *āsana* and off the mat. Over time they will become more aware of when they tend to chest breathe or when they hold their breath. It is hoped that the observational practice will encourage the student's mind to quieten, developing focus and a sense of grounding as they settle into the space. As we observe our natural breath and consequently focus our mind, our breath tends to begin to lengthen.

At this stage, I find it helpful for students who are new to yoga to introduce the idea of inhaling and exhaling through the nose, letting the jaw release and lips and teeth gently part so that the whole face softens. Breathing through the nose can feel strange at first for some students but it will begin to feel more natural with practice. If a student is really struggling with this, I will encourage them to inhale and exhale through both their nose and mouth at first and then move on to focusing on only breathing through the nose when they feel more comfortable.

This can be a good point to focus on lengthening the breath. I ask students to inhale for a count of three or four in their own time, pause for a second and then exhale for the same count. After a gentle pause they repeat the cycle. I like to mention the importance of lengthening the breath, particularly the exhalation, and explain the reasoning behind this in a digestible way! I also mention that ideally they will be able to connect to this calm, steady, even breath through the whole practice. The breath becoming shallow or laboured during the *āsana* is so often a clear sign that the student is pushing himself or herself too far and needs to back off in order to reconnect to their breath and allow it to become the focal point once again.

A useful breathing exercise for particularly anxious students is to ask them to draw their full attention to the exhalation, lengthening it as long as they can. They then pause after the exhalation, allowing the natural inhalation to arrive in its own time. After a pause at the top of the inhalation they then focus purely on the exhalation again and repeat the cycle.

Particularly when the student is in a supine or seated position, you can ask them to begin to focus on breathing into different parts of the rib cage and abdomen. You can introduce them to belly breathing by asking them to start with their hands on their lower abdomen. As they move the hands to the lower ribs you can talk them through the principles of diaphragmatic breathing and then explain chest breathing while they move their fingertips so they are pointing up towards the clavicles. *Āsana* like Child's Pose are a great opportunity to focus on breathing into the back lower lungs as the rib cage expands and contracts. Side bends present an opportunity to breathe more deeply into the sides of the waist, ribcage and armpit area.

I like teaching a simple *prāṇāyāma* with my students before we start the full *āsana*. Inhaling and then exhaling as a group for a count of six and accompanying this with simple movement introduces the idea of the *āsana* being a breath-led practice and can be a powerful way to unite a group of practitioners rather than a series of individuals. During the practice there are so many opportunities to continue to remind the students to use their breath as a guide during the *āsana* practice. Here the breath can help to show us when we are pushing too hard, holding back or finding it hard to let go.

Here is a summary of some ways to approaching introducing breath into a yoga class.

- Observing the natural breath.
- Encouraging inhalation and exhalation through the nose.
- Lengthening the breath, particularly the exhalation.
- Drawing full attention to the exhale.
- Breathing into the lower belly/lower ribs/chest.
- Practising a counted breath practice as a group.
- Using the breath as a guide during the *āsana* practice.

Ujjayi

Ujjayi (pronounced oo-jai) is commonly referred to as 'victorious breath' or 'oceanic breath' and is a breathing technique adopted during the yoga practice that involves gently constricting the glottis within the larynx that we mentioned earlier. The action is similar to steaming up a mirror with a 'haaa' sound to the exhale but the inhale and exhale are both directed though the nose, with the lips and teeth softly closed. The constriction of the glottis speeds up the flow of air entering the lungs encourages deeper passage. The process also gently heats the air due to increased friction. The resonant sound that is produced can be used as a focal point to draw awareness inwards and add a meditative quality to the practice. The vibration in the throat is believed to stimulate the vagus nerve and the baroreceptors with the carotid arteries of the neck that help to regulate blood pressure, although little research has been carried out to prove these hypotheses.

Ujjayi can be adopted at any time on or off the mat. I even find it useful to use *Ujjayi* breath when I am running because it allows me to breathe as efficiently as possible and prevents me from getting a stitch. *Ujjayi* lends itself particularly well to dynamic yoga practices such as Ashtanga Vinyasa yoga or Vinyasa Flow yoga. In Restorative or Yin yoga you may want to adopt a more natural breath that doesn't add such a heating element. A more natural breath might also feel more comfortable during a hot yoga class or during pregnancy.

As students begin to practise using this breathing technique, they can often do so with a little too much force and effort, which can invariably create tension in the body and too much heat. The tell-tale sign is the 'Darth Vader' sound that can be heard at the other side of the room! A good guide is that the student should be able to hear their breath and you too as you pass by them, but no one else in the room should be able to.

Prāṇāyāma

Prāṇāyāma, meaning to regulate or extend the breath or life force, is an incredibly powerful and transformative practice that forms one of the eight limbs of yoga. In this chapter we have already discussed ways to introduce breath into the yoga practice but *prāṇāyāma* is a practice in itself. Different schools of yoga introduce *prāṇāyāma* at different stages in the yoga journey. Integral yoga teaches basic *prāṇāyāma* from day one while the Iyengar yoga approach is to only introduce *prāṇāyāma* once the student is firmly grounded in *āsana*. When it comes to teaching *prāṇāyāma*, I believe that the first step is to only teach what you know and what you regularly practise yourself. When introducing this practice to a student for the first time, encourage them not to strain or put too much effort behind the breath. They should begin to breathe naturally again if they start to feel spaced out, light-headed, ungrounded or anxious. Build up the *prāṇāyāma* practice gradually, just like you would an *āsana* practice.

There are hundreds of different types of *prāṇāyāma*, each with its own particular benefits. *Naḍi Shodhana* (Alternative Nostril Breathing) is a calming *prāṇāyāma* that is believed to balance the right and left hemispheres of our brain. *Kapālabhāti* (Skull Shining Breath) is a cleansing and energising prāṇāyāma. *Shitali* (Cooling Breath) and *Simhasana* (Lion's Breath) both cool the body and release tension, while *Khumbaka* (Retention) helps to increase the vital capacity of our lungs. *Bhramari* (Bee Breath) has a meditative quality and is believed to stimulate the parasympathetic nervous system.

Here is a summary of some of the benefits from practising *prāṇāyāma* regularly.

- The simple action of lengthening the exhalation stimulates the parasympathetic nervous system.
- Breath retention encourages more alveoli in the lungs to open and therefore increases vital capacity.
- Active exhalation helps to recycle the residual volume of the lungs.
- *Prāṇāyāma* develops our internal awareness and has a strong meditative quality.
- In *Āyurveda*, *prāṇāyāma* is used to balance the three *doṣas*: *vata*, *pitta* and *kapha*.

— 3 —

The Art of Composing

'Putting Together' a Sequence

Liz Lark

Vinyāsa krama: step by step, moving towards a special place

I saw the angel in the marble and carved until I set him free.
MICHELANGELO

We come to the mat to practise with ourselves as we are; an act of humility and surrender. We have made a statement: 'Hello Self (or 'selves')! Here I am!' Master teacher Desikachar, who developed Viniyoga, said, 'For an authentic yoga, we explore our entire being in this present moment.' He described how his father, Krishnamacharya, commonly accepted as one of the fathers of modern yoga and who ran a yoga *śālā* (hall) within the Mysore Palace during the 1930s, met his students at the gate, brought them inside to practise and then escorted them back to the gate, demonstrating sequencing beyond the mat. He alluded to climbing a tree in sequencing: 'It is not enough to climb the tree; we must be able to get down too.'[1]

This is an apt analogy for *vinyāsa krama*, literally meaning, 'step by step, moving towards a special place', a central concept of yoga sequencing. The arc of a rainbow describes setting out on a journey with an intention or vision, just as Dorothy in the Wizard of Oz travels along the yellow brick road, meeting obstacles and guides along the way and arriving at the 'Emerald City', reaching the symbolic 'pot of gold', a quality of consciousness or ethereal idea where fear dissipates and truth or being (*satya*) emerges. Her great fear (the wizard) does not actually exist; he is a figment of the imagination! There is peace, integration and resolution at the end of the path as she returns back home and sees it in a new way, with fresh eyes.

The eye altering alters all.
WILLIAM BLAKE[2]

Mental yoga

Within our yoga practice, we set an intention and follow a theme, carving a path to travel in stages towards a peak/apex and then gradually cool down towards rest and resolution, drawing not just a proscenium arch but a full circle, just as we would when hiking a mountain. On the journey we take sips of water, take in the view and assimilate, just as we take a counterpose following a posture, which is rebalancing, gentle and reflective, allowing for bio-feedback (the body speaking to the brain). When we return to the same place, something has changed within us: the process of *śauca* (purification) has cleansed us, a transition from dark space (*duḥkha*) to light space (*sukha*).

The brain can be described as a mountainous terrain, pathways of which have been walked many times, becoming 'fixed' forms of thinking and consolidating habits or beliefs, inherited or otherwise. It is possible to consciously create and trace new 'ghost paths', in the form of ideas or attitudes, which can be walked, trodden and repeated to cultivate and build new neural pathways. This is why mental yoga becomes just as vital as physical yoga as we gently coax the mind towards loving kindness (*metta bhavan*) with the felt sense in the body.

Before we begin to practise, we choose the 'special place' (a *saṅkalpa* or good wish) for integration. Mindfulness teaches that on waking for a new day, it is useful to make a handwritten list to direct the mind on a course through the day and at the end of that day to write a 'gratitude list'. If we do this, we are likely to fulfil these wishes and to rest well. The meaning of *saṅkalpa*, is 'benevolent wish'. As in *Alice in Wonderland*, the magical key fits a small door, and we have to stoop low to get into the castle of yoga. So, first of all, what is our intention?

Create a theme, a thread, that inspires you to weave a path with intention and authenticity.

Visualisation

The soul never thinks without a picture.
ARISTOTLE

The mind needs nourishment in the form of imagination; it is useful to give replenishing, uplifting images during practice. The idea of weaving a silk cocoon as we breathe is one image we may employ. I use the image of a boat on the water to focus on through practice – a metaphor from the *Bhagavad Gītā* for stabilising mind and body to cross the oceans of *saṃsāra*.

Mental intention: *saṅkalpa*

Crystallise your intention for your practice to dedicate the mind towards a path that supports and affirms you and others. This may include the path of *bhakti* (devotion), *karma* (selfless service) and *jñāna* (wisdom, knowledge).

Desikachar said that the 'highest' form of *prāṇāyāma* (yoga breathing) is the natural breath! Invite the breath to permeate three sections of the torso (abdominal, thoracic and clavicular). It is akin to filling a bottle to the brim and then emptying it from top to bottom. We are inviting the mind to become present. When mind follows breath, thoughts become distant.

Metta bhavan means the cultivation of loving kindness. This is an excellent tool to incorporate into yoga sequencing to lay the foundations of *ahimsa* (kindness) and *satya* (truth), the principles of non-violence and clarity that Gandhi lived by in 1930s India, by which he managed to 'smash the system'! *Metta bhavan* begins and ends with self-care and then casts a net out to include others. It is vital to look after yourself first and not selfish to do so (like putting on your breathing mask on a flight, so you can self-regulate and consequently be of benefit to others). It is a mantra (meaning: mind protection): 'May I be well, May I be happy, May I be free from suffering/friction.'

A *saṅkalpa* (good wish) is sown like a seed into the subconscious mind from the outset of a practice and returned to at intervals during counterposes for self-reflection (*svādhyāya* – the second limb of Patañjali's yoga). *Svādhyāya* mirrors the intelligence of supra-personal skills – the ability to self-reflect. This is vital when teaching, in order to cultivate interpersonal skills of kindness and support for others. When psychotherapist Carl Jung was asked, 'Will we make it?' he replied, 'Yes, if we do our inner work.'

Structural sequencing

It is useful to sequence from the 'ground up', from gross to subtle, from outer to inner, starting with the tangibility of body and breath. *Grounding* and *stabilising* connect us to Earth and we become embodied, rooting down like the Banyan tree, the sacred tree of India.

Practice can be structurally anchored in 'hip opening', 'shoulder releasing' or 'core stabilising', which begins your journey from a steady foundation and gives a reference point or coat hanger for targeted creative sequencing.

Be an artist: to quote Maria in *The Sound of Music*, 'Let's start at the very beginning…'[3]

Assemble the pieces and gather inspiration for your *jigsaw puzzle*.

We all need grounding, so we begin practice by connecting with the legs, feet and bones, with hip releases and exploring our bony architecture in relation to gravity. This is best felt lying down, especially as we often arrive at yoga practice having travelled, so a transition to receptive listening mode is welcome to help take our foot off the accelerator pedal – physically, emotionally and mentally. Literally raising our legs over our head can be the best way to shift our energy, in the posture aptly called Active Reversal Pose (*Viparita Karani*), elevating the pelvis on a block, with the legs raised or resting them up a wall. Several minutes of this while reflecting on theme and intention will work wonders to revive us!

Release techniques of contemporary dance are wonderful for helping to connect with the 'felt sense' and to move with sensitivity and literally 'feel it in our bones'. Moving consciously with breathing will start to *recalibrate* the nervous system, inviting us to attune inward, *switch gear*, slowing down our brain waves from beta (active, waking) to alpha (dream state) and even to theta (creative, deep relaxation).

Connect with body and breath

Lying semi-supine is the recommended technique for restoring the natural pulse of cerebral spinal fluid, a subtle energy pulse and moving river through the spine, and the position honours the natural curves in the spine. Tune into abdominal, diaphragmatic breathing felt in the belly, called 'Hara' breathing (this is the Japanese word for belly, considered in the east to be our powerhouse and axis centre of gravity). Recite: 'Inhaling, navel rising; exhaling, navel falling.'

Release technique is a movement practice that focuses on breathing, skeletal alignment, joint articulation, muscle relaxation and the use of gravity and momentum to facilitate efficient movement. It is used in dance and therapeutic movement including Feldenkrais and the Alexander Technique, yoga and martial arts. Dancers at the Trinity Laban Conservatoire of Music and Dance, Greenwich unfold like a flower finding its root channel underground before sprouting upwards. Let us slow down in our exploration of yoga and return to these natural movements, tuning into the felt sense.

To release blocked energy ('grit' or *saṃsāra*) we explore the body-mind landscape to get comfortable in our skin. It is not an intellectual practice nor a competition and it may be a new way of learning and being. Sense the inner landscape of your body, like the sculptural formations of a rock canyon, breathing into the spaces within your joints. Close your eyes if comfortable, so that you can see more (inside).

Invite the breath to slow down, play around with the breath, drinking and digesting it and lengthening the exhalations though the mouth to release spent energy and detoxify. Focusing on the out-breath calms and stabilises the nervous system (*langhana*). The chemicals released will become benevolent endorphins and serotonin, rather than survival, action chemicals of adrenalin and cortisol, which become toxic if over-stimulated.

Pawanmuktasana: 'The yogi's warm up'

To warm up, we weave dynamic and static patterns of movement. We lie either semi-supine (Alexander Technique active rest position: knees bent, feet hip width apart) or straight legs *Savasana*/Corpse Pose. For vulnerable lower backs, supports are included behind the knees and behind the nape of the neck to support the natural curves of the spine.

We loosen and warm the joints with *Pawanmuktasana*, from the traditional school of *Satyananda*/*Sivananda*, in non-weight-bearing rotations, flushing through synovial fluid, another moving river that carries protein and maintains fluid ease.

We know the phrase 'If you don't use it, you lose it'. These are systematic joint freeing limbers, from toes, feet and ankles, to knees, hips, hands, wrists and elbows to shoulders.

Imagine the torso as a flexible rectangle that bends and shapes like the paper fish you find in Chinese crackers that curl up at the corners. Oil and breathe into the corners of the torso, hips and shoulders in the yogi's limber, including rolling your head side to side on the floor, as if it is a glass bowl.

Templates

There is no fixed method for sequencing but we can create templates from which to build a safe practice. The following template of *childhood embryology* is wonderful to follow: honour natural development as a creature flexes (curling inward, protection) and arches (extending and opening). These primary movement reflexes form the first two warm-up movement patterns focused on the spine.

Flexion

The primary embryonic curve is an expression for the inward folding of the spine, like the organic stem of a leaf spine. Somatics practitioners call this the 'Red Light' Pose – when we are drawn in with the front line shortened in a protective stance. In the deep pit of the lower abdomen, a profound muscle crosses the front of the pelvic basin like a swathe sash, or 'energy belt' sheath, which 'bites towards the spine' when engaged, protecting the lower back and stabilising a neutral pelvis. It brings energy and support to the colon, lower organs/gut brain. Fundamentally, this connects us into our 'deep seat', anchoring up psychosomatically (mind and body). We engage this core centre when we exhale and gather the navel and pit of the belly towards the spine. Core work needs to be included in yoga, as it is essential for back stability and mind stability. Following core work, always release with a gentle twist.

Extension

The oppositional stretch to uncurl from flexion. Somatics practitioners call this the 'Green Light' Posture – with extension in the spine, enhanced lumbar and cervical curves, the body weight towards the heels, a tendency towards locked/hyperextension in the knees and spine and chest and chin lifted

There is a third posture, the Trauma Pose, where there may be imbalance between left and right sides of the torso. We use our outer and inner eyes to read the body to address imbalance, seeking a recalibration between 'red light' and 'green light' postures. With great care and kindness (most importantly), we become explorers in our yoga practice as we sequence to rebalance holding patterns (*saṃsāra*).

Examples:

- pelvic tilts
- Cat Pose
- somatic cat stretches (like Cat Pose, but lying semi-supine, arching the spine from the floor on inhale and releasing the spine to neutral on exhale)
- Bridge Flow (*Setu Bandhasana*)
- *Apanasana* (curling up).

Side bending/lateral flexion

Warming and contracting the sides of the waist (the obliques) balances left and right sides of the body brain. The somatic tradition values the contracted side as much as the flexible side – a refreshing take on yoga, which may focus on stretching. Healthy muscles need to be like sponges and shock absorbers so they contract and protect as well as lengthen and release.

Examples:

- Bananasana: supine banana bow stretch, walking all limbs to one side
- Child's Pose, sweeping arms to each side
- Cat Pose with 'C' shape: look back to see your tail, contracting one side and lengthening the other side of the waist
- side-lying somatics (somatics exercises focus on enlivening the somatic centre of the body): start with right side lying Chair

Pose and the top arm loops over head. Inhale, lift the top side of the body, contracting the waist obliques. Simultaneously lift the left lower leg shin, which will contract the lower waist obliques. It might look odd but it is effective triggering for the side waist. Do this five times and then change sides. Release with gentle floor twist.

Twisting/rotation

Twisting/rotation is a complex movement, and the body needs to be prepared for it, so in yoga sequencing, we warm up though this pathway. The hardest pattern to master is rotation – we need to move from our spine and core. Think of an ancient lizard turning his head back – the whole body is involved. The feet need to remain planted as the twist ripples through the entire body, turning the thorax and then the neck after stabilising the core. The tail stays firmly anchored (oh, how I wish we had not lost our tail!).

Examples:

- Butterfly Roll
- Supine Butterfly (*Supta Baddha Konasana*): arms extended out to sides and roll the knees side to side for gentle floor twist.

Balances

Challenging the body to stay balanced and tuning the body in space is called proprioception. All poses develop this ability, waking up muscles and nerve eyes in every cell to become 'awake' and vitalised. All postures are, in fact, balances.

Example:

- Following 'Coffee Press' (symmetrical warm up referred to later in the chapter), shift the weight onto one foot, catch the other knee in the hands. Rainbow sweep the same arm behind you, drawing a rainbow twist balance. Imagine you have a tap root towards Earth, from all four corners of the pelvis (left and right sit bones, pubic bone and tailbone) to tether you to the moment. Transition spinal roll down and release to Willow Tree. Repeat on the other side.

Inversions

Described by Desikachar as topsy-turvy poses, these poses soothe and rebalance us, rebooting our energy.

Example:

- *Viparita Karani*, the Active Reversal Pose, is a wholesome, healing posture for stress and is recommended at the end of each class to soothe and integrate whilst echoing the theme or focus. Lie with the legs up the wall, with a bolster or blocks beneath the pelvis to elevate the lower body. If it is moon time for women, elevate the legs only keeping the pelvis at heart level.

If we balance the six movement groups above, we can achieve a holistic, balanced class, or we can target particular postures for a more energetic or more calming practice.

Practical exercise

Draw an orange on a large piece of paper. Consider the six movement groups and include 'opening warm ups', 'closing relaxation' (bookends), 'meditation/reflection' and '*prāṇāyāma*/breathing'. Divide the orange into segments and create for yourself a 60-minute class, including timings, within each segment. Begin supine (lying) and gradually grow towards standing postures, with smooth transients. In the peak of the practice, add balances to strengthen and any challenging peak pose(s), and then gradually cool down, returning to floor poses, being seated and concluding the class supine.

Preparations and progressions

Warm ups (in the first quarter) progress into stronger, weight-bearing sequences, the archetype of which is the template called *Surya Namaskara*, within which we identify with light as the source of life, with the Sun as our primary source of *prāṇa* and with the sense that we are compressed forms of sunlight. It is an ancient sun worship and crosses ancient cultures and tribes (Aztecs and Egyptians). There are myriad variations of the Sun Salutation, which is fantastic to adapt to your energy or *guṇa*. Originally, mantras were sung during each step of the Sun Salutation, describing qualities of the sun, and were sung in Sanskrit, for example '*mitraye*' means reverence, the one who shines; '*ravaye*' means the one who shines. Poems were recited whilst practising to align oneself with the energy of the Sun.

Seasonal Sun Salutations can be adapted to balance the energy of the season: Ashtanga in winter to warm and invigorate; *Sivananda* in summer to smoothly flow (deep, flowing lunges).

The Moon Salutation is composed of slow, fluid, arching movements, deep lunges and gentle side bends, painting the full moon as we practise. This would suit a calming twilight practice in the evening time.

The Dynamic Sun Salutation of the Ashtanga tradition includes dynamic jumps and challenging *Caturaṅga*, a compelling pose that must be deconstructed for beginners, into *Aṣṭāṅga Namaskāra*, or 'Mini-chat', bending the knees to touch the earth as you lower down from High Plank. Strong, heating, weight-bearing salutations would suit a morning, invigorating practice for those who are fit and able.

The Golden Sun Salutation, for the wisdom years, can incorporate Cat Pose, hands on a chair or wall, with Tabletop Pose (hands on a wall) instead of Dog Pose, for those with high blood pressure, avoiding having the head below the heart.

The Egyptian Salutation, anchored in Horse Pose, does not involve lying prone, so would be good for pregnancy (we can adapt it for pregnancy safety by replacing Cobra with Cat Pose).

Now create your own bespoke sun salutation to balance the dominant *guṇa* (cosmic quality).

Positive effects of posture groups

- Forward bend: calms and cools (*guṇa*/cosmic quality *tamas*) the parasympathetic nervous system. Nourishes the digestive and reproductive systems. Has an exhalation focus to release energy (*apāna vāyu*).
- Backbending: energises and heats the sympathetic nervous system. Balances the thymus (heart), thyroid (throat) and adrenal (root) glands. Has an inhalation focus to invite zest for life (*prāṇa vāyu*).
- Side angle: energises and heats the sympathetic nervous system. Benefits the circulation and respiration. Has an inhalation focus.
- Twisting: has a balancing role. There are both heating twists and cooling twists. Benefits the digestive system and endocrine system and balances the adrenals and thyroid. Same *vṛtti*: an equal inhale and exhale. Balances the nervous system and the enteric nervous system in the solar plexus, which affect digestion and emotions.
- Inversion: calms the parasympathetic nervous system. Soothes and benefits the circulation and pineal, pituitary and thyroid glands. Generally has an exhalation focus. (Note: Head Stand is heating and energising, rebalancing the endocrine, hormonal system. Shoulder Stand is cooling and soothing.)

From the above, we can devise a stimulating daytime practice and a soothing twilight practice. Dynamic repetition is good to warm up the body towards holding static poses to stabilise and strengthen muscles and bones. Dynamic practice can also be 'slow flow', deeply nourishing all '*kośa*' layers. Be mindful that too much repetition can lead to repetitive strain injury (RSI), so vary the sequences. We can also weave a balancing practice that is *sattvic* (vitalising), where we integrate yin and yang sequences. If we painted it, it would look like the peaks and troughs of a cumulus cloud, composed of numerous 'mini-*vinyāsas*'.

Preparations and counterposes for posture groups

Forward bending postures

Extensions of the spine prepare for all poses.

Spinal roll downs, as taught in Pilates, and somatic cat stretches prepare forward bends. Move towards flexion with gentle awareness, tracking the vertebrae like stacking golden coins, oiling the joint spaces as you travel.

CHILD'S POSE

Cat Pose to Child's Pose *vinyāsa*. Inhaling in Cat Pose, arch the spine to extend it. Exhale, consciously rounding the spine into flexion as you breathe out, engaging the deep core muscles and travelling into Child's Pose.

Leg raises from supine using the belt will repair the hamstrings, preparing the hips for flexion.

Counterpose: forward bends with '*Dwi Pada Pitham*', Floor Bridge Pose, slowly elevating the spine into extension, releasing to neutral on exhale. An alternative gentle backbend would be Locust Pose, lying prone (face down) and elevating the chest and heart without hands for assistance – this is a safe backbend that will not agitate the spine and will help to connect to the core centre.

Backbending postures

Warm up with extensions to decompress and do front thigh openers, such as *Virasana*, Hero Pose (sitting with a block under sitting bones to avoid knee strain). Hug the foot behind you for quadriceps stretch or practise low lunge, *Anjaneyasana*, from the traditional Sun Salutation to prepare the hips. Cultivate core connection to protect the lower back (lift pubic bone in lunges). Stabilise the core with pelvic tilts in warm ups. Unlock the shoulders with joint freeing rotations and especially externally rotated, elevated positions such as *Gomukhasana*, the Face of Light Pose (using belt). Gentle side bends will prepare the sides of the spine/torso for backbends. Twists also prepare the spine, wringing it out 'like a wet cloth'.

Do you see how we target the shoulder limbers and hip limbers here for backbending?

Counterpose: these include gentle twists to unwind the spine and forward bends.

Side-bending postures

To prepare the spine for side angles, warm up first with flexion, warming the spine and thoracic extension to target the upper back to release, so that the side angles will be a 'clear colour'. Then develop pathways towards building side angles, always gently at first, like a painter (unless you are Jackson Pollock!). External hip openers will prepare the hips – Reverse Pigeon and Thread Needle.

Example: Bananasana: lying supine and reaching the arms overhead, hold the right wrist with the left hand. Walk both arms and legs to the left side so that you create a 'C' shape, a banana bow, still lying on your back. Breathe and stretch, receiving a healthy stretch and contraction to the sides of the waist (obliques). Feel the oppositional moments complementing each other – as one side extends, the other side contracts, activating and releasing muscles like pistons.

SOMATICS SIDE BEND

Side lying in Chair Pose with bent knees, take the top arm over the head to cup the underside of your face. Inhale and lift the upper torso and head in a side contraction 'C' shape. Exhale and lower the head slowing to de-contract. You can also add the following: inhale and repeat, also elevating the lower leg foot of the top leg, thus contracting the lower waist obliques. This gives a healthy contraction to the top side waist and a lengthening stretch to the underside waist.

Seated: rainbow the arms from side to side in synchrony with your breath.

Counterpose: forward bends gently release the spine following side angles. A gentle twist will release the hips if they have been externally rotated.

Twisting postures

'Extend before you bend': as in all posture groups, extensions prepare twists to decompress, so that the twist is not 'coloured' with flexion and rounding inwards (Red Light Pose). Simple backbends such as Sphinx will prepare the thoracic spine, just as in lateral warm ups. Extending the arms overhead in Raised Mountain will create space. Simple backbends, such as Chair Pose with extension, joint limbers for neck and Rocking Chair will release the spine, rocking forwards into Folding Chair like a willow tree over the legs. Side angles will prepare the torso for twists, balancing right and left sides. Dog Pose will bring deep extension to prepare the spine with space. Do shoulder limber to open the chest and Reverse Kayak limbers to roll the shoulders back and to open the chest and heart in twists.

Counterpose: these release into symmetrical forward bends and gentle backbends to balance the 'red light' and 'green light' postures. Here's where you can discover whether you are more dominant in red or green postures.

Balancing postures

All standing postures prepare for more challenging balances. Make sure you have warmed up the foundation first and prepared the hips with your targeted hip limber to follow the pattern. If it is Dancer Pose, work first on thigh openers as in backbends. If it is Tree Pose, prepare the hips with external rotations and flexion (belt-assisted leg raises).

Counterpose: invite a gentle opposition to rebalance, like a mountain stream, trickling fresh water through the spine – this is usually a forward bend (soften the backs of the knees).

Inversions

All other posture patterns prepare for inversions, but the neck is an alarm point if approaching Shoulder Stand: we are not designed to take the body weight on the neck! Thus, explore alternatives. Prepare a raised platform of four yoga soft blocks, which form a rectangular platform for the shoulders and upper back (Iyengar style), allowing the neck to release and have space. Or elevate the pelvis on a bolster at the wall for *Viparita Karani*, meaning 'active reversal pose'.

Note that a gentle forward bend is an effective counterpose for almost all movement groups to neutralise the body and calm the mind. It is great to use props creatively to assist release.

Weave a silk cocoon

Joy and woe are woven fine
A clothing for the soul divine
Under every grief and pine
Runs a joy in silken twine

——— WILLIAM BLAKE[4]

Cycle of a class: template (cake slices)

The cycle of a class is like walking through the carriages of a train: there is a linear path, but the content and colour within each carriage affects you, recalibrating with each sequence. The cycle is:

- opening
- limbers/warm ups
- Sun Salutations of standing *vinyāsas*
- standing segment
- balancing segment
- backbends
- seated forward bends/hip openers
- inversions
- supported restorative closing sequence
- relaxation
- mindfulness/meditation/reflection/*prāṇāyāma*
- share and depart.

Standing postures

The Ashtanga Vinyasa tradition of Pattabhi Jois describes standing postures as the Mala, Garland or Necklace of Poses, weaving postures like pearls on a necklace.

Group related poses together and then thread them onto your sequencing necklace, moving from simple to more complex postures. Group the postures into open (externally rotated) and closed (internally rotated) hip categories.

If the theme is upper body/shoulders, take specific targeted exercises from the shoulder limber to prepare for your peak poses or equivalent hip limbers on the basis of six movements to oil the ball-and-socket joint.

Have an anchor pose to begin from and return to, like a boat that ventures onto the ocean and then returns back to harbour. There is a wonderful saying in Tai Chi Soft Martial Art, which I carry into the standing sequences: 'Embrace Tiger, Return to Mountain.'

Aim for *seamless choreography* – like a garland of flowers on the thread of silken breath – have the intention for each stage of a pose to be like a smooth, shiny pebble in a *sattvic* stream, which can be stepped upon with each breath to cross the stream.

GROW THE WARRIOR

In sequencing standing poses, aim to practise bent leg poses (i.e. with Warrior foundations) before straight leg poses (e.g. Triangle Pose), which are far more demanding on the legs. Warm up Warrior poses with dynamic repetitions, bending the front knee on exhale and straightening on inhale.

Sample sequence.

- Sun Salutation.
- High Plank.
- Prone.
- Inhale low Cobra.
- Repeat.
- Exhale Prone Crocodile.
- Change sides.
- Swaying Palm Tree.
- Tree Pose.

- Warrior Two.
- Side Angle.

The Warrior can be explored in many ways with alignment. Explore qualities of the Warrior during practice.

STANDING CLOSED HIP SEQUENCE

Breathing mantra: 'Conscious breathing is my anchor.'[5]

Sample sequence:

- Anchor pose: Mountain, Tramline Feet (hip width wide).
- Coffee Press: soften the knees and neutralise the pelvis ('container'). Inhale and sweep the arms skywards, gathering in all *citta vṛtti* (mind stuff). Imagine you are placing it all in a coffee pot. Exhale and press the palms downwards through the mid-line, rinsing through and returning to a bent knee stance (or squat, touching floor with the palms for deeper hip stretch).
- Stabilise the adductors (inner thighs) by bending the knees on the exhale, squeezing a block between the thighs and awakening the pelvic floor. Inhale, tip toe Mountain Pose, training the feet.
- Warrior One, inhale, mobilise in Mountain Pose and then exhale, step the left leg back to High Lunge. Reverse Kayak shoulder rotations and backstroke arms. Spinal twist in Low or High Lunge. Inhale, return to Mountain, hug the left knee to counterpose the hip. Standing Twist. Wrap the right arm around the left knee and rainbow the left arm overhead. Gaze back. Inhale, return to Mountain. Chair/Squat or repeat Coffee Press transition to the second side.

STANDING OPEN HIP SEQUENCE: SIDE ANGLES

Sample sequence:

- High Heeled Lady Dog Pose (lift heels).
- Rotate heels inwards to touch into balletic.
- Exhale squat to Butterfly.
- Repeat. Extend legs to Raised Dog.
- Repeat. Inhale into Pigeon Pose to free the hip. Repeat.
- Level 2/3: add Tail of the Dog, Dog meets Tree, with optional drop over.

Sample sequence:

- 'Greased Lightning hip limber': toes of right foot on the Earth, rock the whole of the leg from the hip joint, oscillating in internal and external rotation to loosen the muscles of the hip (this can relieve sciatica).
- Swaying Palm Tree Pose: place the ball of the right foot outside the left, preliminary stage of Tree Pose, clasp hands over head. Sway side to side in Mountain Pose.
- Level 1: Tree Pose (wall option).
- Optional level 2: Standing Thread Needle (echo floor limber warm up).
- Level 3: Arm Balance, Twisting Variation (*Galavasana*) (preparation shoulder limber in warm ups).

  Counterpose: Weeping Willow Tree, fold forward over hip hinges. Brain Bath.
- Release with standing 'May Pole' spine ascending with soft knees, swinging arms like ribbons around the body in a loosening, warming twist.
- Anchor pose: Horse Pose, Bear Pose (sweep arms up on inhale, opening gesture), Warrior Two, Side Angle, Half Moon,

Triangle, swivel to standing forward bend, rotate to Spinal Twist. Change sides returning to Horse as the anchor pose for the side angles.

Magical transitions: changing gear

Moving from seated to standing, or vice versa, it is important you link each stage (*krama*). Please do not 'just stand up'. Remember you are weaving a silken cocoon on the threads of each breath – keep spinning!

STANDING TRANSITION TO SEATED FLOOR POSES

Sample sequence:

- Anchor pose/*vinyāsa*: Coffee Press to squat. Crane Arm balance (optional).
- Squat Lion Breathing, hands in *Ksepana Mudrā,* clap hands pointing index fingers upwards and making a tower with these two fingers. This *mudrā* (gesture) is said to be detoxifying, inviting Spring energy.
- Squat twist (intestines cleanse).
- Standing forward bend. Or, transition to Seated Cosmic Egg. Boat. East Plank.
- Link three poses smoothly, with breathing: inhale Boat, exhale Cosmic Egg, inhale East Plank, exhale Cosmic Egg. Play and explore the breathing rhythm like a tide to carry you 'across the ocean of *saṃsāra*' (cyclical existence).[6]

Injury can occur when transitions are not mindful or smooth in sequencing, so give particular care to the fluid shifts as we change shape (like Barbapapa, a fictional children's morph-like creature, who changed shape like magic). Motifs from Sun Salutations or Coffee Press can 'bridge the gap', but do not let these be like Polyfilla: honour each mindful step of the jigsaw puzzle with the quality of Zen walking.

CREATIVE TRANSITION

Here is a suggested transition for a core practice focusing on side angles and twists to stimulate the centre of the body (*samāna vāyu*):

- Anchor pose: Forearm Cat. Chisel into thoracic spine, extending (inhale), flexing (exhale) the middle back. Press left forearm alongside the front of the mat. Stabilise by pressing right hand into the mat alongside left hand.
- Inhale, straighten legs out towards High Plank, feet together. Exhale, rock onto the outside edge of your left foot.
- Tilt into Side Forearm Plank Pose. Inhale and lifting the right arm, rainbow sweep the top arm overhead, elevating the pelvis (side bend). Exhale and sweep the top arm hand to the right hip. Rest by lying the pelvis on its side, exhaling.
- Inhale and bend both knees (Side Lying Chair). Exhale, tip upright to seated for seated spinal twist counterpose to wring out the spine.
- Inhale, step the top right leg over the left, planting the right foot to the floor outside the left hip, into *Matsyendrasana*, seated twist. Exhale and engage the navel, turn the spine to the right. Release. Breathe.
- Unspin, pressing the hands to the floor to climb into Dog Pose, walking the legs to release. Lower to Cat Pose. Transition to the second side.
- Following the second side of the seated twist, release the legs forwards into seated staff, *Dandasana*, for forward bend, changing from heated core segment to cooling seated segment of the practice.

Bookend your practice with a meaningful anchor that is authentic to you. It is said that we remember the beginning and end of a sequence most significantly.

Alan Rickman, whom I had the honour to teach, said after class, 'It's good enough for me,' in his unforgettably dry and humorous tone. The practice may be intense, like mining a coal seam, but there is richness, colour and even humour within that intensity. Black is not one tone dimensional: it is a saturation of all colours of the spectrum. Let's practise with the curiosity of a child, bringing humour, colour and joy, whilst mining!

Theme: 'Follow the yellow brick road'

'Allowing the pause' is a winter theme of welcoming rest moments between sequences for bio-feedback for the body to speak to the brain, allowing things to settle and to 'return to source'. On the yellow brick road in The Wizard of Oz, we are given rich material as Dorothy meets the Tin Man, who is in desperate need of oiling, as he is very dry and stiff. What a wonderful basis for a theme! Newcomers to yoga class may feel like the Tin Man; share this image with them with humour. The brave thing is the fact that they have shown up. Scarecrow provides a second theme: he needs a brain! But what kind of thoughts do we invite? This theme could explore the 'rooms' of the mind – the sheath of consciousness called *manomaya kośa* (lower mind, *citta*, means mind stuff). Further along the road, Dorothy meets Lion, who needs a heart to give him courage, another rich theme. It is valuable to deconstruct words as well as postures: strip them down to their roots. The root of the verb 'courage' is French *coeur:* heart. To have Heart. And what about the Emerald City, the colour of the heart and of balance in chromotherapy and *cakra* system? The colour green is said to balance our blood pressure and nervous system. And yet the Emerald City does not exist as a physical place but is clearly a quality of consciousness: *Sat Chit Ananda* (Being, Awareness, Bliss).

Tribal rituals or Zen Koans (minimal poetic phrases) can form a base for themes. The Esalen Indians of the West Coast of California, which is now an inspiring retreat centre, would stand on the bridge facing downstream towards the ocean with the downwards (*apāna*) rushing of the waterfall beneath them. They would breathe out any darkness, any *duḥkha*. Then, facing upstream towards the mountainous source of the waterfall, they would inhale new energy (*prāṇa*, spirit) having released the old. This tradition is practised today and is echoed in the purifying practice Coffee Press, a qigong standing breathing exercise (see page 48).

Theme: cleansing the layers of being, the sheaths of consciousness

A class can invite you to travel from outer to inner being, on the model of five *kośas* – envelopes of being, or layers of consciousness comprising the 'self', which are nourished with the practice of yoga. This can develop into a course developed from a class introducing the idea of the layers (like an onion) of outer body, physical sheath, travelling inwards, sensing the energy body, mind body, intelligence body and bliss body.

1. We begin with *bone strengthening* – *annamaya kośa* (the jacket made of food). Bones protect us; they are our scaffolding housing our vital organs. They are alive, producing vital juice called bone marrow, which manufactures red blood cells, and these protect our immune system.

2. *Prāṇayāma* (energy sheath) *nourished with the breath*: we may explore subtlety in our breathing within sequencing. *Prāṇa* is defined as 'first unit' to 'travel well'. A simple sequence of *krama* breathing in stages, drinking and eating the breath, we flow from Cat Pose to Child's Pose – the mind follows the breath as life force.

   Inhale, Cat Pose. Exhale in three stages: part one – Elbow Cat (forearms touch the floor); part two – hips draw back to heels into Child's Pose; part three – pause. Drop into the gap.

   Repeat several times.

3. *Manomaya kośa: allow the mind to be as it is, without fighting* – mundane, ordinary thoughts. Practice Warrior Sequence, with a mantra to strengthen the mind. Consider the attributes of the warrior, absorbing a story from the *Bhagavad Gītā*. The story of the archer is a noble, inspiring story. It describes the selection of the master archer as the one who sees *just the bird's eye*. He does not see all the details of the surrounding scene; he sees only the target: an illustration of one-pointed awareness.

4. *Vijnanamaya kośa – a door to light*: higher mind and aspiration. Finding the extraordinary within the ordinary, we tap into an aspirational part of ourselves through practice by stepping away from the limited thinking of ego (*ahaṅkāra*) and *citta* (mind stuff, memory, history, herstory). It is useful to imagine the mind as having many rooms or qualities: there is a spacious room free from conditioning called *buddhi*.

   Metta bhavan nourishes this sheath with *saṅkalpa* and affirmation.

5. *Ānandamaya kośa – bliss sheath* – is beyond limitations of conditioning of mind and affectations. This place is where the mind stops: 'Heaven is the place where nothing really happens.'[7]

   Follow the breath so thoughts become distant, keeping the breath and brain away from each other to avoid fanning the fire of thinking (*vṛtti*: rushing whirlpool).

Theme: integrating the eight limbs of yoga

Exploring each limb during practice ensures that we are practising holistic yoga, which includes meditation (limb 7), breathing (limb 4), concentration (limb 6) and *āsana* (limb 3). We know the expression: 'Stop the world, I want to get off!' Yoga is an invitation to do just this, as we step out of linear time (time is 'a calculation of the moments') by absorbing the mind in the creative process where artist merges with object. *Saṃyama*, the top three limbs of Patañjali yoga, weaves together relaxed concentration (*dhāraṇā*), leading to meditation (*dhyāna*), a merging beyond time and conditionings (evenness of mind: *samādhi*).

Weave these concepts into your practice.

Theme: return to nature

Connect with nature and animal kingdoms around you, even if it's a window box, a plant you can grow or a park, to relieve stress and shift perspective away from the human kingdom. Practise outdoors in woodland or by the sea, which lowers blood pressure and gets you out of your head and into your body. Monitor intake of the other kind of 'CATS' – coffee, alcohol, tobacco and sugar – as these play havoc with our balance!

Theme: be a painter: balance light and dark

Honour the pauses. In winter, it is important to tune into the hibernation energy of welcoming darkness, with light rituals of candles and fires, cultivating the '*Hygge*' quality of glimmering warmth and support. We need community for our health on every level; aim to cultivate it. As I write and we wait for 'thawing' and look for snowdrops, we can create a Winter Warrior Practice, which is grounding and heating and strengthening and stabilising, based around the Warrior poses.

Theme: allow things to be as they are

Give yourself this gift of restorative yoga, where you trust the practice to do its work and you step out of the way.

IN ORDER TO INSPIRE, YOU MUST BE INSPIRED

Collect your favourite quotes, song lyrics and stories (contemporary as well as original philosophical primary source material) that provokes an authentic response within you towards *satya* (truth). Share these in your practice and teaching.

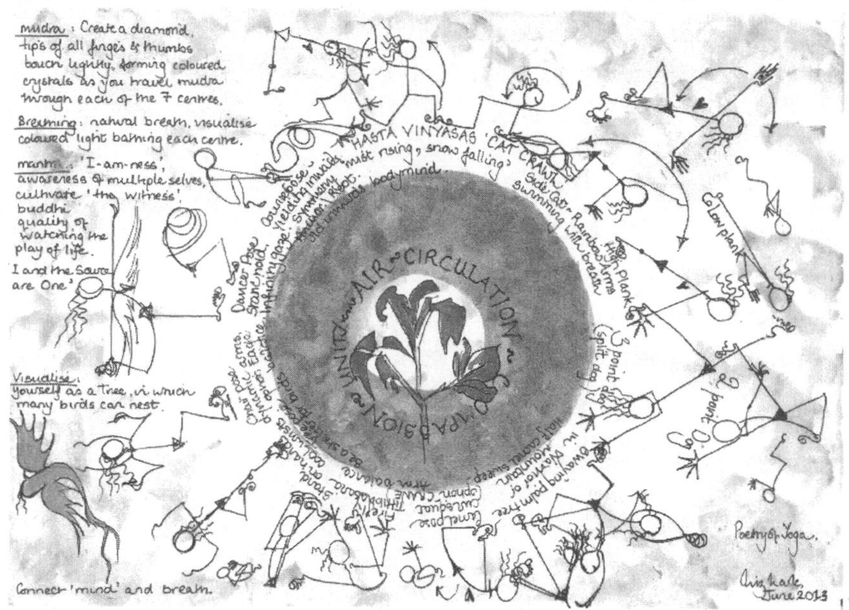

Sequencing towards surrender: a restorative Moon Sequence for stress, with creative use of blocks

- *Supta baddha konasana*: reclining bound angle (Butterfly). Chest and upper back elevated on bolster, facilitating free breathing. Facilitating natural breathing.

  Option: reclining Hero Pose or Fish Pose, depending on knee safety. Chest and spine elevated on bolster. Conscious breathing (arm raises overhead to facilitate breathing space). Hands on lower belly. Shift pelvis on top of bolster, supported Bridge Pose. Open front thighs and lower belly.

- *Viparita Karani*: Active Reversal Pose. Leg raises or both legs up wall

  During these poses: *metta bhavan*, loving kindness affirmation phase one: 'May I be Well.'

Counterpose: *Balasana*, Child's Pose (can hug bolster if comfortable). Forehead resting on block. Hara breathing.

Transition: Cat Pose, slow stretches. Exhale (*langhana*) focus into Child's Pose.

- Floor Yin Twist: sitting 'side saddle', right hip on floor, knees bending in zig zag position (*Bharadvajasana*), right hip touching bolster. Twist torso to lie front of abdomen over line of bolster, releasing as in Child's pose, but with a deep yin twist. Face opposite direction to knees. Do on each side.

- Downward Dog: head resting on high block or blocks. Hands resting on two blocks to open shoulders. Eyes closed if comfortable.

- Yin Pigeon: lying forward over bent leg thigh. For knee issues, lunge instead with hands on two high blocks. Release head forward onto block or bolsters.

- Happy Baby pose or *Apanasana*: knee hugs to chest. Stretching back line.

- Seated forward bends, *Janu Sirsasana*: head to knee pose, forehead on blocks or bolster.

- *Upavistha Konasana*: wide-legged seated forward bends. Head on blocks. Modify bending the knees, sitting on low block or blanket.

- Semi-supine breathing, hands on Hara.

- Relaxation, wrap shawl or sari around the head, gently but firmly and lightly covering the eyes.

- Support the neck with a rolled towel and bolster behind the knees. Warm blanket.

- Guided *Yoga Nidrā*, Rotation of Consciousness. 61 Points/75 Breaths. Ocean breathing.
- Mantra: *Om Saha Na Vavatu.*
- Seated alternate nostril breathing to balance sun and moon, equalising left and right nostrils.

Notes

1 Desikachar, T. K. V. (1995) *The Heart of Yoga: Developing a Personal Practice.* Vermont: Inner Traditions India.

2 Blake, W. (1972) 'The Mental Traveller.' In *The Pickering Manuscript.* New York: Pierpont Morgan Library.

3 Wise, R., Lehman, E., Andrews, J., Plummer, C. *et al.* (2005) *The Sound of Music.* Beverly Hills, CA: Twentieth Century Fox Home Entertainment.

4 Blake, W. and Baskin, L. (1968) *Auguries of Innocence.* New York: Grossman Publishers.

5 Thich Nhat Hanh (1997) *Stepping into Freedom: Rules of Monastic Practice for Novices.* Trans. A Laity. Berkeley, CA: Parallax Press.

6 Eknath, E. (1985) *The Bhagavad Gītā.* Petaluma, CA: Nilgiri Press.

7 Talking Heads (1979) 'Heaven.' *Fear of Music.* Sony/ATV Music Publishing LLC, Warner/Chappell Music, Inc.

— 4 —

Incorporating Philosophy into Yoga Teaching

Graham Burns

Introduction

One of the most misused and misunderstood terms in the yoga world is 'yoga philosophy'. Over many centuries, the practices and techniques that we think of as 'yoga' (*āsana*, *prāṇāyāma*, *bandha*, meditation, etc.) have been harnessed to meet a broad spectrum of philosophical goals – whether that is a realisation of the isolation of 'spirit' from 'matter', a strictly non-dual view of the world as pure being or pure consciousness or a connection to (or even union with) a chosen divinity. As Mallinson and Singleton point out, contrary to the often trumpeted idea that yoga takes the form of 'many paths to a single goal', the reality is that, in yoga, we see a relatively small, and related, number of paths leading to a wide variety of goals.[1]

The first task, then, for any teacher wishing to incorporate philosophical teachings into their classes is to have a clear understanding of the breadth of the yoga tradition(s), to understand that the philosophical viewpoints that underpinned Patañjali's teachings in around the fourth century,[2] with their roots in the dualistic philosophy of *Sāṃkhya* and a liberal sprinkling of Buddhist ideas,[3] are markedly different from those of the strict non-dualist *Advaita Vedānta* tradition a few hundred years later or those of the various, usually theistic, tantric traditions from the last few centuries of the first millennium CE onwards, which (together with ideas from Patañjali and probably from tantric Buddhism) ultimately led to the rise of Hatha yoga around the beginning of the second millennium CE.[4] Although attempts have been made to read Patañjali from an *advaitin* or a tantric perspective, those attempts generally appear forced, as well as anachronistic.

Investigating the various philosophical schools that have harnessed yoga techniques for their own particular doctrinal goals is a complex exercise and not one that I propose to undertake in this chapter (or in an average yoga class!). As yoga teachers, it is much better that we acknowledge and understand these philosophical differences, while at the same time looking for the consistent messages that we can offer our students so that they understand that there is more to yoga than physical exercise. In this chapter, therefore, I look at a small selection of core teachings from the yoga traditions across the ages (which may not be 'philosophical' in a technical sense) that can easily be brought into teaching, and to offer some tips from my own experience on how best this can be done in general classes (as opposed to specialist philosophy classes or workshops).

The essence of yoga

The earliest unambiguous reference to '*yoga*' as a state of being comes in the *Kaṭha Upaniṣad*, from about the fourth century BCE. There, yoga is defined as the steady control (*sthirām dhāraṇām*) of the senses.[5] That control is said to lead the practitioner to a place beyond the distractions of everyday life and, ultimately, to the knowledge of the practitioner's essential self (*ātman*), which, in turn, will free the practitioner from the bondage of the cycles of death and rebirth. As the same text says: 'The creator pierced the openings of the senses outward; therefore one looks outward and not into the self. A wise person, seeking immortality, turned his sight inward and saw his self.'[6]

It is this turning inward, controlling the senses and the mind and getting to know our true self, which is the essence of yoga, whatever philosophical or soteriological implications that knowledge may have for us. As we are all taught in our teacher training (and often before), *Yoga Sūtra* 1.2 describes the state of yoga as *cittavṛtti nirodhaḥ* – the restraint (*nirodhaḥ*) of the spinnings (*vṛtti*) of the mind (*citta*). What we sometimes forget is that Patañjali also gives us a reason for controlling our spinning mind: when the mind is controlled, what Patañjali calls the 'seer' (*draṣṭṛ*) rests in its true essence – in other words, our essential self reveals itself to us (*Sūtra* 1.3).[7] At all other times, we simply get caught up in the spinnings of the mind (*Sūtra* 1.4): we detach ourself from the goal of awareness of our true self because we are worrying about what is for dinner or whether the class is going to overrun and make us late to collect the kids or even whether we are doing *Trikoṇāsana* with 'good alignment'.

If, therefore, we are to bring any philosophical teachings into our everyday classes, our starting point should be to imbue our students with the understanding of this true essence of yoga. I often, not entirely facetiously, say that my introduction to yoga took place on skis, rather than on a yoga mat. For it was when skiing that I first really found myself in a place of complete single-pointed awareness when, for an extended period of time, I was not caught up in my spinning mind. Only many years later, when I stepped onto a yoga mat, did I realise that this state of mind could be accomplished without snow, a trip to the mountains or an expensive lift pass.

However, we should also acknowledge that the process of turning inwards and quietening the spinning mind will be different for everyone. For many of us in the busy 21st-century West, the great starting point that yoga offers is the mindful movement of *āsana* practice. It is unrealistic to expect yoga students to commute from the office to class and move directly into a place of physical stillness, let alone meditation. However, what is important is to convey an understanding that (pleasurable and important though it may be to free the joints and work the muscles) the overall process of yoga is one of moving awareness inward and away from distraction. Our challenge as teachers is not only to explain this to our students, but also to structure the classes that we teach in a way that reflects that inward trajectory. And, if we are truly to be yoga teachers rather than *āsana* teachers, that process should culminate in a period of silent meditation or contemplation.

Stuff

As many yoga students will not tire of reminding you, it is all very well to talk about stilling the spinning mind, and getting to know the self, but stuff constantly gets in the way. Rather than simply shrugging our shoulders at the inevitability of this, how can we answer our students within the framework of the teachings of yoga? *Yoga Sūtra* 1.30 lists nine 'impediments' (*antarāya*) to the path: illness (*vyādhi*); idleness (*styāna* – more literally 'density'); doubt (*saṃśaya*); carelessness (*pramāda*); sloth (*ālasya*); intemperance (*avirati*); false understanding (*bhrānti darśana*); ungroundedness (*alabdha bhūmikatva*); instability (*anavasthitatva*). At some level, most of us will probably be impacted by most of these at some stage: sickness will prevent us practising; doubt will set in, perhaps about whether we are practising the right style of yoga or whether the practice is 'working'; we will prefer to stay in bed rather than get up to practise; we will intemperately push too hard and then beat ourselves up for carelessly injuring ourselves. And so on.

As teachers, it can be valuable to remind our students (and ourselves) that these impediments are not 'new' products of our contemporary age (however much that may exacerbate them) but that they were acknowledged right back in one of the seminal texts of yoga. Sometimes – though not always – their causes may lie in the five *kleśas* or 'afflictions' (rather a loaded word: 'obstacles' might be a better everyday translation) listed in *Sūtra* 2.3 – ignorance (*avidyā*), egoism (*asmitā*), attachment (*raga*), aversion (*dveṣa*) and clinging to life (*abhiniveśa*). Of these, *avidyā* is said, in *Sūtra* 2.4, to be the 'field' (*kṣetra*) or breeding ground, of the others and is defined in *Sūtra* 2.5 as 'seeing the non-eternal, impure, and sorrowful non-self as the eternal, pure, and joyful self.' This brings us back to the essence of yoga: as a result of this lack of understanding of our true nature, perhaps through over-identification with our constantly changing physical body, our sense of ego drives us to attachment and/or aversion. In other words, we get caught up in the impermanent impediments and become miserable, when joy lies in recognising the impermanence – we will (in most cases) recover from our illness, our doubts will resolve, our lethargy will dissipate, etc. – and replacing it with an awareness of the eternal and essentially joyful true self.

This can be a useful message to bring to students both generally and in one-to-one situations. When we see a class of students practising intemperately, perhaps striving too hard to 'achieve' a particular posture, we can offer a gentle reminder about the impediment of intemperance and the obstacle of attachment. And don't forget that the opposite can also apply – if we see a class of students practising slothfully, sometimes a reminder about the obstacle of aversion can work wonders! So, when stuff arises, can we, with compassion, meet our students with the knowledge that, according to the teachings of Patañjali, these things will pass if we devote ourselves to appropriate practice? As Patañjali says in *Sūtra* 2.11, 'the spinnings of the mind produced by these obstacles are eliminated by meditation' (*dhyānaheyās tadvṛttayaḥ*)

I am not (just) my body

Although not mentioned explicitly in any yoga texts until the 17th century,[8] the idea that the individual is made up of a series of interconnected layers – usually referred to as *kośas* or sheaths – appears implicitly to inform the processes of yoga, whether the 'eight-limbed' model of the *Yoga Sūtra*,[9] with its progression from the so-called 'external' limbs to the 'internal' limbs, or the various models of Hatha yoga, with their progression through, for example, cleansing techniques, *āsana*, *mudrā/bandha*, *pratyāhāra*, *prāṇāyāma*, and stages of meditation, such as *dhyāna* and *samādhi*.[10]

The *kośas* first appear in the *Taittirīya Upaniṣad*, probably from around the sixth century BCE, where they are described as five identically shaped 'bodies', each located directly within the previous one. The outermost is the body consisting of the 'essence of food' (i.e. the physical body) or *anna(rasa)maya*, followed by the bodies consisting of *prāṇa* (*prāṇamaya*), the cognitive mind or *manas* (*manomaya*), intelligence (*vijñānamaya*) and bliss (*ānandamaya*).[11] As a model of the human make-up, they can be very profitably used in teaching as a way of explaining the yogic progression from the outermost physical layer (manifested primarily in *āsana*), through the layer of *prāṇa* (impacted by *āsana* but more directly by *prāṇāyāma*, *mudrā* and *bandha*) to – and beyond – the mental layers accessed both through meditation and, to an extent, through practices such as *Yoga Nidrā*, as well as in how we take our yoga 'off the mat' and into our daily life. Their relevance in contemporary yoga is well demonstrated by their use as the organisational template for B.K.S. Iyengar's 2005 book *Light on Life*.[12]

The various layers all interact with each other. As T.K.V. Desikachar said, 'The first step of our yoga practice is to consciously link breath and body.'[13] And we all instinctively know that the state of our breathing and the state of our mind are directly related. Most of us will teach breath-linked movement as a staple of our teaching, yet sometimes as yoga teachers we become so attuned to reminding our students simply to 'breathe' in *āsana* practice that we forget to teach them how, via the relationship of breath and mind – or *prāṇamaya*, *manomaya* and *vijñānamaya* layers – different breathing patterns can have different effects on the way that their mind will respond. Above all, we should remember *Haṭha Yoga Pradīpikā* 2.2: 'When the breath is unsteady, the mind is unsteady. When the breath is steady, the mind is steady, and the yogi becomes steady.'

Understanding this make-up of the human person is also important for those who have studied in tantric yoga traditions and wish to bring into teaching some of the complex tantric models of the body that influenced the practices of Hatha yoga from the early second millennium CE. Those models generally revolve around the movement of *prāṇa* through an extensive network of channels (*naḍī*), with the flows of *prāṇa* being subject to blockage at certain points (*granthi*) and concentration at others (*marma*). The way in which *prāṇa* moves, or is concentrated, is directly affected, according to Hatha yoga, by yogic practice, while, at the same time, the control of *prāṇa* leads to the control of the mind, which remains the ultimate goal of Hatha yoga. Additionally, numerous different models developed of a system of *cakras* – or 'wheels' – as focal points for meditation along the body's central vertical axis or *suṣumnā*. It is not the place of this chapter to explore these varied ideas of the tantric yoga body in any detail (Mallinson and Singleton (2017) contains a good summary of them at pages 171–183) but simply to note that judicious introduction of them (if properly explained) into teaching can also enhance a student's experience of himself or herself as more than just their gross physical form.

The slow fix

We are conditioned in our modern lives to expect instant responses and results. Students are disappointed when they cannot touch their toes in their second class or affronted when you politely point out that attendance at an intermediate class presupposes more than just a couple of beginners' classes. But yoga is not a quick fix. The *Yoga Sūtras* make clear that we are in it for the long term. As *Sūtra* 1.12 explains, the control or restraint of the spinning mind requires practice (*abhyāsa* – literally 'application of oneself') coupled with dispassion (*vairāgya* – literally 'lack of excitement'). As Georg Feuerstein has pointed out:

> Practice without dispassion is conducive to an abnormal ego-inflation…and thus entanglement in things worldly. Dispassion without practice…is like a blunt knife; the

> psychosomatic energies generated through the turning away from mundane objects remain without an outlet and at best cause confusion in body and mind.'[14]

That practice – the effort (*yatna*) to gain stability (*sthiti*) in the control of the spinning mind[15] – requires, according to *Sūtra* 1.14, proper cultivation, without interruption, for a long time. For the contemporary student, it requires going to the appropriate classes, attending class regularly, developing a self-practice and (perhaps above all) neither expecting a quick fix nor beating themselves up when the bind in the twist is out of reach. As teachers, it is our role to explain to our students that they have signed up for a programme that might take longer than one meagre lifetime, one that is implicit in the word '*yoga*' itself, which is much more accurately translated as 'discipline' than 'union'. At the same time, if we practise with awareness, each step on the journey can be important – and enjoyable.

Being awake

We have seen that part of the essence of yoga is getting to know our real self. But how can we do that if our yoga practice drifts onto automatic pilot? All of the *yamas* and *niyamas*, both those in *Yoga Sūtras* 2.30–45 and the extended lists found in some recensions of the *Haṭha Yoga Pradīpikā* and elsewhere,[16] can be usefully employed in yoga teaching, but perhaps one of the most important in the contemporary yoga world is *svādhyāya*. Literally, this means 'self study', which is usually taken in contemporary yoga to mean study of the self, though older interpretations tend to suggest that it means study of scriptures 'appropriate to oneself'.[17] Either is appropriate, for, as Bryant points out, most ancient Indian philosophical scriptures contained teachings about the self.[18]

While *Yoga Sūtra* 2.44 describes the result of *svādhyāya* as 'union' (*samprayoga*) with one's chosen deity, such an overtly theistic result need not be part of contemporary yoga teaching – especially as Patañjali himself plays down the theistic side of yoga. The '*Vyāsa*' commentary[19] gives the rather more practical result of *svādhyāya* as the fulfilment of the practitioner's wishes. More important for our present purposes is the idea of study *of* the self, not necessarily at a deep metaphysical level, but at the everyday level of exploring the effects of practice on our own physical body, breath and mind. As yoga teachers, we have a duty to encourage our students to approach their yoga practice with a constant sense of enquiry. What impact does, for example, a strong backbend practice have at a physical, energetic or emotional level? If a certain posture or practice causes discomfort (at any level), how do we manage that discomfort, perhaps through modifying or even ceasing the practice completely? This is not to make the practice too 'heady' or analytical but, rather, to emphasise the importance of developing a sense of deep knowingness and understanding in our practice: a Sanskrit word often used in this context is *buddhi*, a word with several meanings, but perhaps most effectively translated as 'presence of mind' (and deriving from the Sanskrit root *budh-* , meaning 'to wake up'). If we can encourage our students to stay awake in their practice, not only are they more likely to stay safe, but we can also encourage them to move towards the *niyama* of *santoṣa* – contentment – which *Sūtra* 2.42 teaches leads to 'unsurpassed happiness' (*anuttama sukha*).

Balance and equanimity

The *Haṭha Yoga Pradīpikā*, from around the 15th century CE, gives us a list of six behaviours that cause the state of yoga to be 'utterly lost' and six that are conducive to success in yoga. The first six, in *Pradīpikā* 1.15, are over-eating (and/or possibly under-eating), over-exertion, too much talking, performing unnecessary austerities, socialising and restlessness. The second six, in *Pradīpikā* 1.16, are enthusiasm, open-mindedness, courage, knowledge of the truth, determination and solitude. We are often taught that yoga practice is not competitive, should not involve pushing to the point of strain and so on, yet many of us will have been to classes where the ethos appears to be the exact opposite. We have probably also been to classes that feel more like social meetings than deep individual practices. What these lists of behaviours emphasise is that yoga is not about extremism in any direction but is rather about finding a 'middle path'.

The *Bhagavad Gītā*[20] describes many different approaches to yoga, not just the four that are commonly trotted out (*Karma* yoga, *Jñāna* yoga, *Bhakti* yoga, *Rāja* yoga). One of the most useful in teaching is the description of yoga as 'equanimity' (*samatva*).[21] It is worth remembering too that the *Yoga Sūtra* uses similar language in describing the result of practising *āsana* with the harmony of steadiness (*sthiratva*) and comfort (*sukhatva*) – one becomes unassailable by opposite forces (*dvandva*), such as pain and pleasure, heat and cold, etc.[22] While the idea of equanimity follows nicely from the idea of non-attachment (*vairāgya*) to the results of practice – which is, of course, also a key teaching of the *Bhagavad Gītā* – *Sūtra* 1.33 gives us some specific guidelines in particular situations: 'From an attitude of friendliness towards the happy, compassion towards the suffering, joy towards the virtuous, and equanimity towards the wicked, comes calm in the mind.'

From moment to moment, most of us can switch between these four states, even in our yoga practice. We can be happy one moment when everything seems to be flowing smoothly without distraction and suffering the next for any one of the many reasons we have already discussed; we can be virtuously practising one week and embracing 'wickedness' by pushing too hard, annoying our neighbour or forgetting to turn our phone off in class (the ultimate yogic wickedness!) the next week. As teachers, can we embody these four attitudes (borrowed from Buddhist teaching, where they are known as the *brahmavihāras*) in our own behaviour and encourage our students to do the same? Or, in the terms of the *Haṭha Yoga Pradīpikā*, can we encourage in our students a balance between enthusiasm for yoga and the courage to deepen their practice, on the one hand, and not striving too hard or no self-mortification on the other? As holders of the space in the yoga studio, can we encourage social conversation to take place after class rather than immediately before or during?

A sacred space

In the world of yoga mats routinely costing over £100 each,[23] it is easy to question the need for a rectangular piece of rubberised (or more eco-friendly) material on which to practise. But the ancient texts make clear that, if we are to move our awareness inward and beyond distraction, we should practise in a suitably conducive environment. The *Śvetāśvatara Upaniṣad*, perhaps from the third century BCE, teaches that one should practise yoga in a place that is 'level, clean, free from pebbles, fire and sand…not offensive to the eye and…sheltered from the wind'.[24] Over a millennium and a half later, the *Haṭha Yoga Pradīpikā* calls on the practitioner to practise in a secluded hut that is moderately proportioned, 'well plastered with cow dung, clean and free of insects'.[25]

As teachers, we can encourage our students to make their yoga mats – whether costing £20 or £120 – their sacred space, their symbolic cow dung plastered floor. This involves treating our yoga mat, and that of others, with respect: keeping it clean – it is gratifying that many yoga studios now provide mat cleaning materials; putting it away neatly at the end of class; not stepping on someone else's mat if that can be avoided, etc. It can also be a helpful – and perhaps light-hearted – way of encouraging students to bring their focus onto their mat, especially if there are external distractions, for example the music coming from the adjoining studio or the noise of traffic outside. For the hour or two of class, encourage your students to see the mat as their sanctuary – and their laboratory – on which to explore their connection to their self.

A final *OṂ*

If you choose to chant *OṂ* in your classes, how much do you explain to your students its meaning and symbolism? *OṂ* has been a symbol of the absolute – however that may be conceived – in India since ancient times.[26] The *Kaṭha Upaniṣad* describes it as leading to wish fulfilment,[27] and other ancient Indian texts, including the *Chāndogya Upaniṣad*[28] and the *Bhagavad Gītā*, teach that chanting *OṂ* at death can lead to heaven or at least to a propitious rebirth.[29]

Patañjali brings *OṂ* (also known as the *praṇava*) firmly into the yoga context in *Sūtras* 1.27 to 1.29, where he refers to it as the symbol of *īśvara* (the lord), and explains that its recitation in a meditative state of mind is conducive both to turning the mind inward (*pratyakcetanā*) and to the disappearance of the impediments to yoga that he sets out in *Sūtra* 1.30. So perhaps, at least every now and again, consider explaining this to your class as a way of anchoring the chant into the ancient teachings and bringing your students back to that essence of yoga?

Some practical tips

So, having decided which aspects of philosophy you would like to bring into your teaching, how do you approach that task in a way that will be accessible to your students? Here are a few practical ideas.

- As with all yoga teaching, it is important to meet your students where they are. Some students will love to hear more about the philosophical ideas of yoga; others will (to begin with, at least) simply want to stretch their hamstrings. Don't expect everyone to understand, let alone relate to, what you are saying – and, of course, in the spirit of *Sūtra* 1.33, show compassion to those who might be suffering in their effort to take it on board.

- Introduce ideas in lay language before introducing complex terminology. For example, talk about the 'self' before introducing the term *ātman*. If you use Sanskrit terms, explain them unless you are absolutely certain that your students understand what you are talking about.

- Have a clear intention. What exactly are you trying to convey? Try to convey it in a way that is true to the spirit of the teaching, even if you don't directly cite texts or use Sanskrit terminology.

Often, a reasonable paraphrase of a teaching can be more accessible than a strictly accurate translation.

- Try not to confuse teachings from different sources and traditions too much. Yes, the yoga traditions over the centuries have influenced each other, but try to understand the origins of what you are teaching; this will aid your understanding, and, as a result, that of your students.

- Similarly, try to be consistent or, at least, explain any inconsistencies. If you present one idea one week and an opposing idea the next – which might be a perfectly valid thing to do – remember to explain why you are doing this. Otherwise, students are likely to come away confused (and/or think you don't know what you are talking about!).

- Keep it simple. One or two ideas per class clearly expressed is better than a number of ideas that are confused, inconsistent or poorly explained.

- Finally – and importantly – use philosophical ideas as pegs on which to hang your class sequencing. For example, if you choose to talk about balance and equanimity, consider which practices might both challenge your students' equanimity and encourage it, and structure your class accordingly.

Ultimately, whether, and to what extent, you bring the more philosophical teachings of yoga into your teaching is up to you. But, from a set of traditions as deep and as rich as the varied traditions of yoga through the centuries, it seems a shame if, as teachers, we ignore them completely. Perhaps the final – and most liberating – teaching that you can give your students is that which Patañjali gives us about stilling the mental spinnings in *Yoga Sūtra* 1.39: *yathā abhimata dhyānādva*, which we can loosely translate as 'or meditate on whatever you like'.

Notes

1 Mallinson, J. and Singleton, M. (2017) *Roots of Yoga*. London: Penguin. p.396.

2 A date of fourth to early fifth centuries of the Common Era (CE) is now widely accepted as the likely date of compilation of the *Yoga Sūtra* and its most famous commentary, that attributed to '*Vyāsa*' (literally 'the compiler'), which, it has been persuasively argued, may in fact been compiled as a single text. See Maas, P. (2013) *A Concise Historiography of Classical Yoga Philosophy* In Franco (ed.) *Periodization and Historiography of Indian Philosophy*. Vienna: Publications of the De Nobili Research Library. pp.53–90.

3 For more on the overlaps between the teachings of the *Yoga Sūtra* and Buddhism, see de la Vallée Poussin, L. (1937) 'Le Bouddhisme et le Yoga de Patañjali.' *Mélanges Chinois et Bouddhiques*. Brussels: Institut Belge des Hautes Études Chinoises. pp.223–242.

4 Although generally broadly influenced by tantric ideas, Hatha yoga texts normally have relatively little strict philosophical content, focusing rather on techniques. However, there are exceptions: e.g. the *Gheraṇḍa Saṃhitā*, probably from the 18th century, shows a clear *advaitin* bent (see Mallinson, J. (2004) *The Gheraṇḍa Saṃhitā*. Woodstock: YogaVidya. p.xiv).

5 *Kaṭha Upaniṣad* 6.11. All translations from Sanskrit are the author's.

6 *Kaṭha Upaniṣad* 4.1.

7 The different schools of Indian philosophy use different terms for this self, as well as having different understandings about its nature and relationship (if any) to the wider world. The most commonly used term is probably *ātman*, but teachings with a relation to *Sāṃkhya* philosophy often prefer *puruṣa*. *Draṣṭṛ* may be used in *Sūtra* 1.3 as a more doctrinally neutral term. Irrespective of the philosophical school involved, the general principles of *Sūtras* 1.2–1.4 speak to the essence of yoga as a way of practice.

8 Mallinson and Singleton 2017, p.184.

9 *Yoga Sūtra* 2.28–3.8.

10 This is the path set out in the *Gheraṇḍa Saṃhitā*. Other Hatha yoga texts show similar inwardly moving trajectories of practice.

11 *Taittirīya Upaniṣad* 2.2–2.5. The Sanskrit suffix *-maya* simply means 'made of'. In some later Indian philosophical schools, the layers were presented as coverings of the self, but this is not explicitly stated in the *Taittirīya Upaniṣad*.

12 And for Rama, S.; Ballentine, R., and Ajaya, S. (1976) *Yoga and Psychotherapy*. Honesdale: Himalayan Institute Press.

13 Desikachar, T. K. V. (1995) *The Heart of Yoga*. Rochester: Inner Traditions International. p.19.

14 Feuerstein, G. (1979) *The Yoga-Sūtra of Patañjali*. Rochester: Inner Traditions International. p.34.

15 *Yoga Sūtra* 1.13.

16 See, for example, the sources at pages 79–85 of Mallinson and Singleton 2017.

17 In the '*Vyāsa*' commentary on *Yoga Sūtra* 2.32, *svādhyāya* is explained as study of the scriptures and the repetition of *OṂ*.

18 Bryant, E. (2009) *The Yoga Sūtras of Patañjali*. New York: North Point Press. p.273.

19 See note 2 above.

20 The dating of which is widely debated but is probably somewhere between about 200 BCE and 200 CE.

21 *Bhagavad Gītā* 2.48.

22 *Sūtra* 2.48.

23 Or even more: Baller Yoga offer a leather mat priced at USD 1000.

24 *Śvetāśvatara Upaniṣad* 2.10.

25 *Haṭha Yoga Pradīpikā* 1.14. There are similar teachings in other texts. Note that cow dung has antiseptic properties.

26 Feuerstein (1979, p.44) suggests that 'The humming of *oṃ* is in fact one of the oldest and most widely practised techniques of Yoga.'

27 *Kaṭha Upaniṣad* 2.16.

28 Probably from around the seventh or eighth century BCE.

29 See also Mallinson and Singleton 2017, p.260.

— 5 —

Once Upon a Time…

Yoga and Mythology

Tanja Mickwitz

I think most of us love a good story. In fact, modern-day philosopher Jason Silva goes so far as to say that what differentiates us on this planet is that we are a storytelling species. This is how we both make meaning and understand it. For as long as I can remember, I have had a sense that there must be an underlying thread to my life. For many years, I seemed to have this knowing even though I truly could neither see nor understand how it was weaving its way through. Then, at some stage, the stories seemed to emerge more clearly; I started to have an understanding of the unfolding of events and how they related to each other. I started to appreciate how dark times had been initiations, challenges had provided the growth I needed and unexpected turns had led me exactly where I needed to be. This was, of course, an evolution of understanding that came in conjunction with my discovery of yoga and the deepening of my practices. Connecting to witness consciousness gives us clarity to decipher, decode and deconstruct our patterns and behaviours in a different way. This is also what enables us to make different choices – or write a different story, as it were. It is an integral part of the growth process to be willing to examine the stories we tell ourselves and which stories we decide to believe. The stories we choose to identify with are what shape us and determine our experience of life. A story can give perspective and act as a reflection of ourselves.

My foray into teaching mythology naturally started with a story. I had got hold of *The Myths of the Asanas* by Alanna Kaivalya and I absolutely loved getting some background to the exotic names of the poses. It made me realise that what I knew so far had only been scratching the surface of this vast tradition. In fact, this is still the case. The more I learn, the more I realise how little I know and that even in a lifetime it is only possible to learn a sliver of all this rich tradition has to offer. Reading Kaivalya's book, I loved how now the *āsana* came to life more with a background story.

The story of Astavakra

One pose and story that particularly captured my imagination was that of the sage Astavakra. The story goes that even before he was born and was still in his mother's womb, Astavakra was an adept of the *Vedas*. His father was also a lover of reciting the *Vedas* but unfortunately his Sanskrit pronunciation was terrible. As Astavakra listened to his father's less than perfect Sanskrit whilst still in the womb, he couldn't help but begin to shout out corrections. As you can imagine, his father was less than pleased with being corrected by his yet-to-be-born child. In the end, he got so irritated and enraged that he shouted out and cursed Astavakra that he would be born with every bone in his body broken. Harsh indeed, but then many of the old tales tend to be. So this is how Astavakra got his name. Astavakra means eight angles, referring to the deformed shape he was born with due to having so many broken bones. But Astavakra was a born seeker and he cared little for his physical challenges or outer appearance. From being a young child, he studied the science of yoga and the Vedic texts. As he grew into a young man, he kept hearing rumours of an enlightened king called Janaka who held court for many sages and the seers in his court. Astavakra felt that this was where he needed to go – to this place where he could sit in the company of wise teachers and continue to learn from them. So he set off on the very long (and, for his physically challenged body, arduous) journey through forests and mountains to reach Janaka's kingdom. It took him several days and nights, and by the time he reached the palace he was both exhausted and excited. He walked up the steps to the palace and as he entered the gates to the courtyard he saw all the wise men gathered in satsang. One of the sages turned and looked at him, then another turned around, and soon all the men had turned around. One of them pointed at Astavakra's disfigured shape and soon they all began to point and laugh. Suddenly Astavakra fell to the ground and seemed to be shrieking with laughter, indeed the loudest of them all, which made the rest stop and King Janaka walk up to him. Janaka exclaimed 'Who are you? And why are *you* laughing?' Astavakra looked up at Janaka, tears streaming down his face. 'I'm not laughing, I'm crying. I'm crying because I made this long journey. I came so far hoping to find wise teachers, and all I've found is a bunch of shoe-makers,' he sobbed. 'Shoe-makers?' Janaka enquired rather offended, 'What do you mean? We're not shoe-makers!' 'Yes, you are – all you're doing is looking at the skin – judging it to be good skin, bad skin... you have no desire to look beyond the surface or find the truth of what's on the inside.' And in that moment Janaka realised his big mistake and how this young man in front of him was indeed wiser and more learned than any of them. And so it came to be that Astavakra became King Janaka's teacher and a revered sage.

I love this story because it illustrates so well how true yoga really is an internal journey. In a world where we get so overwhelmed by visual impressions of yoga via social media, this story is an especially good reminder of what the practice really is about. So this was the first story I told in class, where naturally I sequenced towards *Astavakrasana* as the peak pose. And not only did the students really enjoy the element of storytelling, but also I realised that I really enjoyed teaching this way – offering the story as a way to add yoga philosophy to the practice.

The next step in using mythology came when I taught a retreat and decided to focus on four of the Goddesses; four aspects of Shakti. And with this came the realisation that there was so much more depth to the practice when invoking the different qualities of the devis. Storytelling adds a certain flavour, but we can choose how deep we take it. It can remain fairly superficial and simply add some entertainment value. But we can also use it to really invite a deep dive into the soul. How do we relate to the archetypes and events on the deepest level? How do we recognise ourselves within the story and what can we learn from it? This is what keeps me interested personally, where we are willing to meet the edge of transformation and begin to tell the stories of our own lives in a different way.

The power of archetypes and symbolism

Looking at archetypes is an incredibly useful way to get a feel for human traits and qualities in a clearer way. Archetypes transcend purely intellectual understanding; through imagery and stories they speak to us in a way that connects all the way to soul and spirit. Using the archetypes of Indian deities in teaching is clearly not an invitation to deity worship. It isn't about invoking something outside ourselves. The deities all hold aspects of our (divinely) human nature and as we invoke them we are simply invoking and igniting parts ourselves that are already present to a larger or lesser extent. It can be incredibly useful to name parts of ourselves in this way. The imagery and full sense of a deity and their qualities can give an immediate sense of what is happening or needs to happen. This sense connects on all levels. There is an immediate physical, emotional, mental, energetic, spiritual response once we have some familiarity with a deity. For instance, if you know you have to summon up the courage to speak up for something you know is unjust, then invoking Durga will be useful. Instead of just thinking, 'I need to be strong, I need to be courageous,' you now have the whole physical and energetic sense of this goddess, riding her tiger, with eight arms with various weapons to cut through to the truth and face the battles you need to face. When we are familiar with these archetypes, they speak to us in a fully integrated way; we feel it through all the layers of our being rather than just relate to it on a mental or intellectual level.

Indian mythology is a good way to incorporate yogic philosophy. As you delve into the stories a little more, it quickly becomes clear that the same story can be told from many different perspectives depending on tradition or philosophy. I suggest always telling stories from a deeply anchored personal understanding; this is what prepares the ground for engaging storytelling that will land with listeners.

So where do we even begin? The Indian pantheon can be confusing, to say the least. Who are these deities and how do they relate to each other? There is really no one answer. The characters pop up at different places in scriptures and stories. And the same story often comes in many variations with different emphases and twists and turns. I have found the following map useful to organise it in my own mind; this is from a tantric perspective. I look at it as a kind of family tree, but let's remember a map is only a map and not the actual reality. So all of which I'm about to describe of course exists within each other. At the top of the tree we have Param Shiva, the ultimate reality (not to be confused with Shiva in his formed form as a deity). Then we drop down one step and we have Shiva and Shakti. Here, Shiva is the pure consciousness of the universe and Shakti is the creative force of the universe. From this level, the universe begins to take form and then we drop one level to the main deities in charge of the universe. Here we have Brahma as the creator, Vishnu who sustains the balance of the universe and Shiva in his form as the destroyer. So you can see that this really is the cycle of beginning, sustenance and dissolution that is at the core of everything in the manifest world. In this realm we also find Shakti in her many forms as Saraswati who helps Brahma organise the universe, Lakshmi as unconditional love who is Vishnu's consort and then Parvati who is Shiva's partner and in her more fierce forms becomes Durga and Kali. The level below this is the heavenly realm where we find Indra as the King of the Gods and the other Gods such as Surya/the sun, Vayu/the wind, Yama/death and so on. Here we also find many demons, of course. This could be equated to our conscious mind and the different pulls within it. And then, finally, there is the world, with humans in it, and at times the main Gods take human form. They came down as avatars, like Vishnu taking the form of Krishna to restore the balance of the universe.

Bringing teaching to life with mythology

I always think of creating and teaching a class as how you might approach a painting. You might start in pencil sketching an outline, then begin adding colour gradually, adding depth of perspective, tone and even texture. The more experienced you are as a teacher, the more nuance and layers you will be able to add skilfully. If you choose to use a story or a deity as the theme of your class, this will be the seed from which everything else grows. A good starting point is to distil down what the main quality, trait, action or feeling is that you intend to invoke. You could call this the '*bhav*', the feeling intention, of the class. A good way to anchor your theme is to come up with a theme title of no more than three words that incorporates the *bhav* of your class. From there you can decide on the appropriate group of *āsana* to focus on – how can you best embody the *bhav*? You now have the broad sketch, and from here you can begin to colour, adding *mudrās*, mantra, subtle body energetics, *prāṇāyāma*, meditation and maybe a suitable playlist if you use music and start getting into the quality of language you want to use. If you tell a story, you can get creative in using parts of your sequence to illustrate parts of the story, and in your *āsana* you can embody the iconography and symbols to really anchor the intended *bhav*.

To illustrate one approach, I will use the following template. I like to think of it as a lotus flower, with the theme of the deity and *bhav* in the middle and then how it is expanded into a class as the different petals of the lotus. You might choose to simplify and just concentrate on a couple of the petals or you might feel comfortable embracing several 'layers'.

- Deity/story + *bhav* = theme.
- *Āsana* – apex pose(s).
- Energetic focus: chakra/element/*vāyu*.
- *Mudrās*.

- Mantra.
- *Prāṇāyāma.*
- Meditation.
- Language – thinking of key words that reinforce the *bhav*.
- Key symbols – how these can be embodied within the *āsana*.

An example using Ganesha's symbolism, iconography and story

Ganesha is the much-loved, elephant-headed, Lord of Wisdom, and also known as Vighneswara, Lord of Obstacles. Not only is he the energy that helps remove obstacles in our path, but he is also the placer of obstacles; in other words, he gives us the opportunity to grow through challenges. He is the son of Shiva and Shakti (in the form of Parvati). Ganesha relates to the root chakra; he is in his very physicality the embodiment of steadiness. His big elephant ears symbolise the capacity for listening and his small eyes show the gaze turning more inwards. In one hand he has a bowl of laddoos (Indian sweets) symbolising the sweetness of life. He has one hand in the gesture of '*Abhaya Mudrā*' for 'fear not'. He carries a sword for discernment and a noose, which could be for the ability to pull things close or as a way to reign in focus. His trunk represents the *kundalini shakti* and also the twists and turns of life. His trunk reaches for the sweets, just like the *kundalini shakti* moves towards the ultimate sweetness of finding the Self. It is said that his big belly holds both the whole of the universe (all we need is already within us!) and the *Agni*, the fire of transformation.

Let's now look at how we can now craft a class around Ganesha applying these principles. Ganesha has this quality of steadiness and he stands at the threshold of new beginnings. So the theme could be to ground into this moment, the threshold of now. The next step is to think about how we would cultivate this quality, this *bhav*, in the *āsana* practice. There are, of course, several pathways you could choose, but if we begin by looking at the energetic quality, we know that Ganesha relates to the first chakra and the element of earth is naturally the most stabilising. In terms of the *vāyus* we would want to connect to *apāna*, the downwards movement of *prāṇa*. This naturally leads on to forward folds, and you might want to have a specific focus on standing poses for stability and grounding. There is also the element of fire with Ganesha carrying the *Agni* in his big belly, so there could be an element of twisting. Twists are good preparation for forward folds and they also have a stabilising effect energetically. So what in the symbolism of Ganesha speaks to this *bhav* of grounding? We have the small eyes for turning attention inwards and the big ears for deep listening. There is the nose for drawing the concentration in to this moment and then, of course, we have the laddoos as the sweetness of being fully present in the now. From the beginning of the practice you could introduce *prāṇāyāma* of *sama vṛtti*, even inhale and exhale, to cultivate both the steadiness and the presence. And, of course, the ultimate practice of fully being in the moment is meditation. Guiding students into a variation of witness meditation practising the steady body could be a way of continuing to use the symbolism of the big ears and small eyes.

- Deity: Ganesha.
- *Bhav*: Stability.
- Theme: Ground with Ganesha.
- *Āsana*: Standing poses, hip openers.
- Energetic focus: *Muladhara* chakra – *apāna vāyu*.
- Mantra: *Om Gam Ganapataye Namaha – Gam*.
- *Mudrā*: Ganesha *Mudrā*, *Abhaya Mudrā*.
- *Prāṇāyāma*: *Sama vṛtti* – stability.
- Meditation: *Kaya Sthira* (Body Steady) and witness meditation.

There are many wonderful stories about Ganesha, but for the sake of simplicity I will here use a fairly short story and then concentrate on some of the iconography to illustrate one example of how you could build this into a class.

> Once upon a time Ganesha was travelling home through the forest on his vehicle, the little mouse known as Moosika. The path through the forest was lit by the full moon, which at this moment in time was always full. Ganesha felt very happy and content; he had enjoyed an evening of joyful festivities and eaten large amounts of his favourite laddoos, the delicious Indian sweets, and his big belly was full. All of a sudden, a snake slithered across the path and and startled Moosika. The poor mouse came to a sudden halt and shrieked, and Ganesha tumbled off Moosika's back onto the ground and his big belly burst open and all the sweets fell out. As you can imagine, this looked rather comical and Chandra, the moon, couldn't help but laugh uncontrollably up in the sky. Ganesha, on the other hand, was less amused and his embarrassment turned into quick rage. He broke off one of his tusks and hurled it at the moon whilst cursing him: 'I curse you – how dare you laugh at me – you will never shine again!' And so it was that the whole world turned dark at night. Can you imagine a world without moonlight? Not only was it dark, but night-time lost its moonlit magic that inspires both romance and poetry. People stopped going out after dark because the paths were no longer lit up and they didn't feel safe. The poets lacked the inspiration they normally got from the moon shining beautifully and eventually they stopped writing altogether. In the end, the Gods realised they had to do something as the world continued to plunge into deeper darkness in all ways. They called Ganesha to a meeting and pleaded with him to remove his curse. Ganesha did realise he'd acted rather rashly, but as he still felt the sting of embarrassment he agreed the moon could shine again but only half the time. This is why we

now have the cycle of the moon, which of course is an absolute necessity in devising the cycles of nature, growth and tides. And later, much later, Ganesha came to use his broken tusk to write down the *Mahabharata* as the scribe for Vyasa. And so it is that what may seem broken can become our greatest gift and 'curses become verses'; this is the path of true transformation.

There are some obvious elements in the story that can be used creatively. There is the moon, which we can embody in some lunar salutations and then naturally *Ardha Candrāsana*, the half moon perfectly symbolising the initiation of the moon cycles. *Bhujangasana* can take on the role of the snake in the story. All the twists and movements of the spine can be a continuous anchoring point into the change of perspective of how the path is not always clear and how challenges can be turned into the greatest blessings. Tightness and resistance give us the gift of exploring a deeper breath for example. And Elephant's Trunk Pose (*Eka Hasta Bhujasana*) could be a natural apex pose, naturally because of the name but also because it requires the activation of the fire in the belly and a willingness to transform and face the challenge.

- Story: Ganesha and the Moon.
- *Bhav*: Facing the challenges.
- Theme: Obstacles into blessings.
- *Āsana*: Twists as symbolic of the twists and turns of the story, twisting perspective. Apex pose: Elephant's Trunk Pose/*Eka Hasta Bhujasana.*
- Energetic focus: *Manipura* chakra – Fire of Transformation.
- *Mudrā*: Ganesha *Mudrā*, *Agni Mudrā.*
- *Prāṇāyāma*: *Kapālabhāti.*
- Meditation: Meditation on the fire at the navel centre.

Let your creativity flow!

You can really have a lot of fun getting creative using *āsana*, *mudrā* and a combination of the two to illustrate points of a story or the iconography of a deity. It becomes the playground for your own imagination. If you decide to use a story, you can choose to tell the story at the beginning of class and then refer back to it during the practice. You could also tell the story through the class, however this obviously requires the ability to hold focus in several different places at once, as you need to be able to weave in sequence, alignment points and adjustments whilst still remembering the story and where you are within it. In my experience, both work well and you can make students feel that they are 'in the story' through both these gateways. I believe that what's important is that you really connect to what you want to get the embodied experience of – this returns to the *bhav* and theme of your class. In the beginning, keep it as simple as possible. You don't want to overload yourself with too many things to remember, nor do you want to overload your students with too much information to process. More detail will come as you become more comfortable and familiar with the material. The more it becomes a part of you, the more you'll be able to share in a way that can be received fully.

I will share a few ideas I have used in the past to get you started; however, these can be expanded on in an infinite number of ways. One recurring theme is the lotus, which in itself carries so much symbolism of the yogic journey – moving from dark muddy waters towards purity and light. Lakshmi rises out of the cosmic ocean on a lotus and many deities have a lotus in one of their hands as a symbol of the spiritual path. You can sequence a whole class around the lotus with *Padmasana* as a peak pose. I have used this whilst telling the story of Lakshmi in the past. You could also use *Padma Mudrā* as an anchoring point to keep returning to in your sequence as you add it to different *āsana*. *Mudrās* are great to use creatively in this way and I highly recommend you get a good book on *mudrās* (they would require their own chapter here). Being energetic seals, *mudrās* are great to use both for meditation and dynamically within *āsana*. In addition, they are often symbolic, which fits so well with theming in mythology.

Many of the deities have weapons in their hands and there are often battles involved in the stories. The *Vīrabhadrāsana* or Warrior series of poses are, of course, a good illustration for how we embody the warrior spirit. Virabhadra is the fierce fighter created by Shiva in his rage. The poses in themselves are already powerful, but you can have some fun with adding variations to the arms such as circling and cutting through the air like an axe or creating a sword with both arms together. In *Vīrabhadrāsana III* you can even feel your whole body become a sword. In fact, many *āsana* lend themselves to this kind of play when you start to explore feeling and form from the inside out.

If there is fire in the iconography or there are *tapasya* practices within the story, this is a great reference to use in the more dynamic parts of a practice when the heat is rising in the body. Of course, the real fire of transformation is more psychic than physical; the mental element of practice is where deep change takes place. To connect to the fire, you can also use *prāṇāyāma* practices such as *kapālabhāti* or meditation on the fire at the navel centre, as suggested previously in the example with Ganesha.

Mala beads often appear as a symbol of mantra and meditation. I sometimes think of the whole *āsana* practice being strung together by the breath like beads on a mala. In addition to *Malasana* or Garland Pose, there are also poses that in their shape can become like a garland, such as *Nataraja* and *Chapasana*/Sugar Bow variations in other poses like *Ardha Candrāsana*. These could also illustrate Ganesha's noose, of course. Really, it's just about inviting your imagination to play!

In the end…

The examples I have given you are really just meant to be a little taste of what is possible, to serve as ideas to get you started. The most important thing, as with all teaching, is that you decide to use mythology because it is something that really resonates and holds meaning for you. There are so many stories and so many variations of the stories, which gives you, as the mythopoetic storyteller, a lot of licence to give your own personal interpretation and understanding. But there also needs to be relevant reason for using this backdrop to teach to; there needs to be something of value to students that reaches beyond the story, beyond the mat and into their lives. Most of all, it needs to be authentic to you. One of my teachers, Yogarupa Rod Stryker, once said that really most of what you teach is who you are. It is the transmission of your connection to your inner truth that will have the most impact on students. And this can be conveyed in so many ways in our teaching; for some of us it feels really natural to speak the language of myths and stories, whereas for others it will take a different form and language. What matters is that it is true to you.

— 6 —

Yoga and Language

Antonia Boyle

Brief introduction to neuro-linguistic programming (NLP)

Neuro-linguistic programming (NLP) was created in the US in the 1970s by two academics, Richard Bandler, a mathematician, and John Grinder, a linguist, as a way of identifying how successful people were able to excel in their various fields including business, therapy, sport, arts, communication and many others. They were curious to know what it was that really made the difference between good and excellent performance. They began by studying (or modelling) three therapists.

Bandler and Grinder found that even though these therapists each worked differently, they all possessed remarkable abilities of building *rapport*. Bandler and Grinder 'modelled' their subjects' exquisite rapport-building skills and by doing this were able to replicate, more or less, the same results. As they developed the model, now known as NLP, along with co-developers like Robert Dilts, they discovered a number of *pre-suppositions* or *beliefs* that now underpin this powerful system.

So that you can begin to use these valuable techniques and principles in your teaching, without the need to become a fully fledged practitioner, I will introduce you to a few of these *pre-suppositions* and how to apply them.

The efficacy of NLP relies on its ability to guide people through the 'how' to do something, rather than just the what is happening or going wrong. Many people already understand what the problem is, but they don't know or can't see a way to change it.

NLP simultaneously looks at what can go wrong while building rapport and offers the how-to skills to make changes.

How to build and maintain rapport with a group

So what exactly is 'rapport'? When asked, people give mixed answers: being on the same wavelength, feeling understood, being listened to, being afforded a sense of trust and respect, etc. None of the answers is wrong, but it's not always easy to pinpoint exactly what happens when people are in rapport, until you start to analyse in it in practice.

Observing small groups of people in rapport is very revealing.

- They sit/stand in similar ways (e.g. legs crossed, arms crossed, leaning forward/backward).
- When one person moves to a different position, the whole group moves bit by bit.
- Breathing rates, tone of voice and speed of speech are similar.
- There are many more similarities.

Pacing/matching and leading

Pacing (or matching) is an important component of building rapport. It involves entering the other person's model of the world, so you begin to behave like them. You match your students' *unconscious* sense of what is real for them. They can then relax and trust in the feeling that they are understood and feel safe in that knowledge.

In this instance, *unconscious* means they are not consciously aware of the process; they just get a general feeling that what you are providing is exactly what they need, that you have understood them and that they trust you.

Once rapport is established you can start to lead your students to where you want them to go. As yoga tutors, we all want our students to leave class feeling better than when they walked in.

Rapport = Influence

Example of pacing/matching and extreme mismatching

Imagine taking a small child for a walk. You hold their hand and you match their little footsteps. You are pacing the child and all is well. The child won't *consciously* know you are doing this on purpose. However, *unconsciously*, the child is contented because you are matching the child's capabilities at that time (i.e. small steps), which is their own reality.

After a while, the going is far too slow, so you start taking larger steps. In no time, you end up pulling the child along, who is now screaming! You mismatched the child's sense of reality and what it means for them to go for a walk – the rapport was broken with negative results.

The above scenario represents the what, not the how.

Number 1 Presupposition: the map is not the territory

This means that we all create a map of our own inner world. This map is totally unique to each individual and is our reality; it expresses what is true and real for us. Our 'map' is not usually the 'true map' for someone else, even when we *believe* that we fully understand another person, we can only *presume* that we really know someone else's inner world.

We all create our own reality based on a set of beliefs gathered throughout our lifetime. These might be beliefs formed early in our life or learned somewhere along the line from direct experience. Often, the beliefs formed in early life are those of our parents/carers/influential adults, which we hold onto, even if they don't serve us well. Whatever we learned from an experience resulted in a set of beliefs. Beliefs can change, but the real power of a belief is that it is always true to the person it belongs to – these beliefs form the basis of the rules we live our lives by. Beliefs can be limiting or resourceful.

People usually need evidence to change a belief. If you make statements to students that do not match their reality at the level of their beliefs, they find it difficult to relate to these statements and mismatching occurs, resulting in loss of rapport.

However, positive and resourceful belief-change is possible. I demonstrate an example of this during my NLP for Yoga Tutors course, with a technique that enables students to undertake or go further into a difficult posture that they thought was beyond them.

This powerful demonstration shows that common sense and reasoning alone do not always lead a group to believe that something is possible for them. However, when NLP is introduced, a positive change to limiting beliefs can occur and seeing this in action clearly demonstrates the outcome.

The demo

Before I begin, students warm up for *Hanumanasana* (the Splits).

I then establish who can do the Splits (99% say they can't). I ask them to show me how far they can go. They believe they can't possibly do this. This is called their Present State.

My outcome is to enable them to change their belief, so that they can either go deeper into the stretch or just believe it is possible to go deeper by practising. This would be their Desired State. In this case, it's not necessarily about being able to do the full posture but for the group to know that, with practice, they might be able to do more.

For the Desired State to be achieved they will have to hear, see or feel something that resonates with them so that they get a sense of the possibility for achieving more.

For me to say, 'Of course you can do it; all of you can do it!' would be a total mismatch for the group's beliefs, and any rapport I might have made would be lost. So I am *matching* and *pacing* their reality by asking them to see what might be possible right now. This is called *leading*. I am leading them gently towards the idea that something might be possible now. Because I had already established and maintained good rapport with the group, it was safe for me to 'presume' and lead. When they do the posture again, many can go deeper into the stretch or believe that it 'might' be possible, because they have been given permission to see how much might be possible right now. I did not tell them that they would go further into the posture, but I invited them to just see what might be possible right now.

This is a very gentle way of leading. I am giving them the choice to 'just see if it might be possible'.

Number 2 Presupposition: you have within you all the resources you need to achieve what you want to

This NLP belief relates to the fact that we don't need to *add* anything to ourselves – we are already perfect. We have all the resources within ourselves – we just need to learn how to access and engage our inner resources. All we need do is remove whatever holds us back from revealing our perfection. This is totally aligned with yoga, as we practise postures to remove stiffness and let our natural flexibility see the light. We relax to remove the effects of stress and allow our innate tranquillity to shine through. We don't have to add anything at all. We simply uncover our perfect self.

It is very common for some students to volunteer that they were able to do the splits when younger (but not anymore). I ask one of these students if I can demonstrate how they still possess the resources they had back then. They might just have forgotten how to access these inner resources and it might not be related to being older! Remember, a belief is a rule we live our life by. If you believe that something is possible then the opposite is also true!

Exercise

This exercise will allow you to get a sense of pacing and leading, as well as underpinning the NLP Number 2 Presupposition (above). As explained, this resonates with the ultimate goal of yoga – to find our inner perfection.

When I do this, I position it as a bit of fun to the class and the volunteer. I'll ask the volunteer to come up to the front, but give her permission to stop the exercise at any time if she finds it uncomfortable. She will be assured that this is not a 'test' for *Hanumanasana*! She will not have to talk, unless I ask a question. While we have this conversation, I match her body positioning and breathing as much as I can.

Once we start the exercise, I stand slightly behind and just out of sight behind her right shoulder. It ensures I'm not 'in her face' and enables the volunteer to think and remember without distraction.

Finding inner resources on the timeline

- Ask the student to imagine a line on the floor running from the Present, where she is standing to the Past (behind her) and towards the Future (in front). This is her timeline.
- As the student is now standing in the Present and facing the Future, ask the student to do the posture in that place, so that we have an idea of how much she can do right now, i.e. the Present State.
- Ask the student how old she was when she was able to do the posture.
- Instruct the student to walk backwards on the imaginary timeline to the time when she was that earlier age. Gently touch her shoulder to support the backwards walk.

- Once she arrives at that earlier age on the timeline, ask the student what inner resources she has that enable her to do the Splits. (Speak in the present as though you are speaking to the younger person.)
- The student will give examples of inner resources, such as: a sense of fun, wanting to be the best, just knowing that she could do it, being flexible and liking to be the best.
- Encourage her to fully remember what it feels like to have these resources and feel them now. What does she see? What does she hear? How does it feel?
- As she mentions these inner resources one at the time, repeat them to her as you touch her shoulder.*
- Ask her to walk forward on her timeline to the Present, while you hold her shoulder gently.
- Once she arrives at the Present, suggest that she turns round towards her younger self and imagines that the younger self is sending her all these inner resources. Mention them to her one at a time. Watch her receive the inner resources and keep your touch on her shoulder.
- Ask the student to carefully do *Hanumanasana* again. She might be much nearer to the floor this time or it may be obvious that she now believes it is possible for her to learn to do the posture.
- Ask her to walk into the future on her timeline and stop at any time in the future she feels is right – it could be 10, 20 or even 50 years from now.
- Ask her to turn around, and point and say: 'Look at the you over there standing in the Present, and send her any wisdom, any resources, anything the Present you could

do with right now! Anything the future you has gathered over time. Take your time. You don't have to say these words aloud.'

- When finished, walk the student back to the Present, and get her to do the posture again.
- It will be clear that she can move much deeper into the posture than she believed possible before.
- Once she has done that and you are still touching her shoulder, tell her: 'At any time in the Future when you might be stuck on anything at all, you can ask yourself: "Was there ever a time when I could do this or something like this? How did I manage that? What resources did I have available then? How can I use these resources now?"'
- Finish by asking the whole class to attempt the posture again – many of them will be surprised by how much more they can do, simply because they have been mentally processing what the volunteer did for herself, even if they have never even tried the pose before!

*The touch on her shoulder is called 'anchoring'. This should be done when the student feels good about something. The touch 'installs' an anchor or trigger. Each time she needs to get back to that same positive feeling again, all she needs to do is touch her shoulder and the feeling returns.

Note: I've used the female pronoun for convenience only.

How to make use of these principles in normal teaching

Be creative! If I'm working with a group on backbends and want them to attempt *Chakrasana* (Wheel Pose), I know many will struggle! I ask them to lie on their backs, close their eyes and relax. I ask them to take themselves back to when they were younger and routinely did exercises as part of playing. I'll say something like:

> Remember a time when you were much younger, and you might have been just playing at doing this exercise. You might have called it the 'Crab'. And even if you never did it yourself, I would like you to remember maybe seeing others doing this. Once you have this picture of the posture in your mind, imagine or remember the ease and lightness you felt in your body when you did this – the fun – and imagine what it would feel like to just take a deep breath in and on the out-breath just push up into the posture! And *now*...place your hands on the floor by your shoulders, take a deep breath and come into the pose.

This is an example of how I 'model young children'. By imagining their inner resources – endless learning without inner soul-searching and excuses of why something is not possible! Young children are the fastest learners. In their first year, they learn a language of sorts – how to psychologically manipulate situations so that they get what they need, how to get up from lying down to standing on both feet, etc. Modelling children allows us to model a sense of adventure, capacity for fun, strong willpower and a drive to learn new things.

Your students will be willing to play: to be a child again. This will only happen if you have rapport with them. Often, adults forget what inner resources they have. If they did not have these resources, they would not have survived life. Having a go and pretending to be child-like often creates leverage in non-resourceful beliefs, and with leverage comes possibilities!

Meditation and relaxation

When I finished my formal NLP training, I explored the possibilities of applying it to all areas of my personal life and professional work. Subsequently, I used my knowledge of NLP and combined it with meditation and relaxation techniques (based on NLP principles) to discover easy ways of helping people to find stillness and relaxation in a matter of minutes. I developed this learning further and began training individuals and groups in the practice of meditation and relaxation.

During my NLP training, I remember one of my trainers explaining how important it was to have rapport with ourselves. If our goals were not in accordance with our unconscious mind and beliefs, it would be extremely difficult, if not impossible, to succeed. In fact, we would be out of rapport with ourselves, creating internal conflict.

Students and clients often tell me that they can't empty their minds. This statement is absolutely true. It is the nature of our mind to be active and observe the world around us and then process it so that we make sense of it. To fight this natural state of the mind creates inner conflict and gives us reasons to beat ourselves up, and in the process of doing this we lose rapport with ourselves.

To progress my ideas, I decided to model subjects who are adept at taking their minds to an altered state – young children. They were often very busy, but suddenly just stopped and stared into space with a relaxed jaw and a very light breath. When I asked the children, 'What were you thinking about?', they usually said, 'Nothing,' or 'Don't know.'

After observing how young children are able to just move into this slightly altered state, it became obvious that by 'widening' their visual view, i.e. seeing peripherally, their brains slowed down and became still.

Because modelling excellence is one of the foundations of NLP, I modelled (copied) these children and used the findings to create a sequence for finding stillness through meditation.

As humans, we experience our world through our senses – our neurology. For the purpose of this exercise we will just deal with seeing (visual), hearing (auditory) and feeling (kinaesthetic). Usually one sense is more developed than another. But when you teach a group, it's best to make use of the three main senses to ensure you include all students, irrespective of their dominant sense. This increases a sense of rapport with everyone in the class, no matter what their individual unconscious preference of neurological sense is.

THE STEPS TO A QUIET MIND

Step 1: Seeing

- Sit down comfortably. Bring your arms out straight in front of you, palms and thumbs lightly touching. Arms are relaxed at shoulder height. Hands are a little higher up so that when you look to your hands you can focus your eyes on the little V-shape that you are making with your thumbs at the top of the thumbs where they touch each other.
- Slowly start moving your arms sideways but keep looking straight ahead as if the V-shape is still there. Without moving your head or eyes, you can still see your arms and hands moving to the sides. Keep looking straight ahead. As soon as your arms are out of sight, drop them down and into your lap.
- Keep looking ahead and lightly to each side too, as if you can still see your hands there. Your eyes will become defocused and you will have peripheral vision.
- Stay like that for a while. It is fine to blink and even to close your eyes gently, as long as you can feel the relaxed muscles in your eyes and still have this sense of the peripheral.
- If you lose that contact with the relaxed eyes, open the eyes and establish peripheral vision again.

This is a useful exercise to practise a few times as a first step with a group.

Step 2: Hearing

To reduce chattering in the brain, loosen your jaw. When you think and have internal conversations, you will move your jaw muscles. People who talk to themselves a lot, move their jaw a lot! You can often see their lips move. They may not be aware of this. Do the following to stop or reduce internal chattering.

- Do the visual peripheral vision exercises and then close your eyes.
- Relax your jaw; let it drop.
- Bring the tip of the tongue to the roof of the mouth, just behind the front top teeth.
- Notice the sound around you (add your suggestions, such as: the sound of breathing, a ticking clock, movement in the group, noises outside, etc.).
- If at any time your attention drifts away from the sounds around you, gently bring your attention back to any sound you can hear.

Step 3: Seeing, feeling, hearing

After taking the steps above, do the following.

- Defocus your eyes as in Step 1.
- Notice your hands resting on your body.
- Feel the different parts of your body that touch the floor/chair.
- Feel the movement of your breath.
- Listen to any sounds you might hear outside.

- Listen to your thoughts – continue to listen as if you are an observer. Just notice them.
- If at any time you forget to listen, just take your attention back to your thoughts.
- Listen in a detached way.

You will find that you will have thoughts, and you will notice them. Rather than forcefully trying to still your mind, accept the thoughts for what they are: your mind is processing its realities. The difference between trying to stop thinking and just observing the thoughts will be that you will be surprised by how few thoughts you have. You will be in control of your thoughts and not the other way round.

The pink elephant syndrome! Stating in the positive

What does 'stating in the positive' actually mean?

When you instruct a group (yoga or any other), it is important that you tell them what you want them to do or experience and not what you don't want them to do or experience. The unconscious mind can't negate. Just look at the statement below and see if you can do what it asks of you – give yourself a moment to do the following:

> I don't want you to think of a pink elephant with yellow spots on its back, especially not if there is a monkey on its back banging cymbals together.

I bet you could not stop yourself from seeing this pink elephant?

Remember, when you are teaching, you are in a position of authority, whether you like it or not. You are very influential (if you have good rapport!) and this means that your students will try to follow your instructions to the letter. If you were to instruct them, for example, on how to do a balance such as *Vrksasana* (Tree Posture), you could say the following:

> You are going to do the Tree Pose in a moment and what you must *not* do is lose your balance. It is very difficult to stand on one leg. *Don't* worry if you feel wobbly; whatever you do, *don't* worry.

Just read this again and then leave out the italic words. Can you see what the unconscious hears? So asking people to *not worry will get them worried.*

Saying to a group that something is difficult sets them up for having a difficult time. Say 'This is *not* easy.' The unconscious will lose the 'not' and will hear 'This *is* easy.'

Ask for what you want rather than what you don't want: some examples

Only install positives.

'This is not easy'

Use the following sentences in class:

- Just imagine being able to feel that 'lightness' in your body.
- Feel how rooted you are to the ground (balances).
- Picture yourself doing this easily.

Be patient and start introducing this over time – it really takes time

To state in the positive does not mean you are not saying something negative. You can still state in the positive, regardless of whether the intention is beneficial or negative. But of course, we are only concerned with positive outcomes here! If you tell a person not to lock their knees, you are protecting their knees, which is very positive. However if you hear yourself say the words *not* or *don't*, then think to yourself, 'I don't want her to lock her knees; what do I want her to do?' The answer would be something like, 'Keep your knees soft.'

If you are stuck for the words to 'state in the positive' just ask yourself the question, 'I don't want this or that; what do I want instead?' and you will have the answer.

What is the function of the unconscious mind?

- It does not process negatives. Use 'This is less easy,' when you want to say that something is going to be difficult. Say 'Relax' instead of 'Let go of tension.'
- It stores memory.
- It organises all memory within its own time and space frame and triggers.
- It represses memories with *unresolved* negative emotions.
- It presents repressed memories for 'rationalisation'.
- It may keep the repressed emotions repressed for protection.
- It runs the body. It has a blueprint of the body in perfect health.
- It receives and transmits perceptions to the conscious mind when appropriate.
- It maintains instincts and generates habits.
- It uses and responds to patterns, symbols and metaphors.

Relaxation

When I began incorporating NLP into my classes, I had to write out all of my relaxation scripts. This was because I was so used to stating in the negative, such as, 'Don't be tense,' etc. Now I find it really hard to state in the negative and have to think what that might be! Once this method started to filter through into my teaching, students remarked on how deeply they would get into their relaxation practice. I didn't explain what was different, but it was great feedback for me. I'd also begun to pay attention to pacing and leading at that time. In my two-day NLP for Yoga Tutors course, I apply the foundations of NLP to teaching yoga. This includes 'how to do your relaxation session NLP style'!

There are many yoga, meditation and relaxation teachers who do not use or are not aware of the principles of NLP. This is not to denigrate their methods at all, but I have a strong belief that adding NLP to teaching greatly enhances the experience and the outcome.

Guided relaxation: the steps

- The process to follow is pace, pace, pace and lead. Pace, pace, lead. Pace, lead, etc. Pacing is to enter the other person's map of reality/their world. Only tell them what they *really know* to be true. For example, 'You are lying on the floor, your feet are touching the ground, your back is touching the floor.' Leading is to get them to where you want them to go. For example: 'And now you can relax.'

- Only state in the positive.

- Use metaphors when you want them to have a certain experience. For example, if you want them to feel secure: 'Solid as a rock' or 'Be fully supported by the floor.' For optimism, 'As sure as day follows night' or 'The outlook is bright.' Just be creative!

- Plan a script just as you would plan a lesson. What are your aims and objectives? How are you going to satisfy these aims and objectives, i.e. what are you going to do or say?
- Have an introductory period with lots of *pacing* – to build rapport.
- Make sure you sit down on the floor to pace their physical state as much as possible. This will also affect your breathing and your relaxed state. Your energetic state is going to be similar to theirs too.
- Have a *leading period* when you take them to whatever outcome you have in mind for them.
- Before you bring them back, do *future pacing*. This is telling them what they can expect when they come out of the relaxation and for the rest of the week or even longer.
- When you bring them back to now, tell them that they will be completely aware and back with you in the present.

The bare bones of a relaxation script

Lie down on the floor, making sure that you are comfortable. As you are lying there, you can begin to become aware of your body. Know that at any given time, if you feel you need to move, that is fine. And as you lie there getting ready to be completely relaxed, it is important for you to know that from time to time it is possible to be aware of sounds, either inside or outside this building. These sounds may be noticed, although they don't seem to have anything to do with your relaxation. You can make these sounds work for you, so that each time you hear a sound you will feel that you relax even more, even deeper. *(This is a 'command' and a lead for the future, for something that is not happening yet. This is called a 'future pace and lead'.)*

As you sink into a deep relaxation you will stay awake and aware, and even if your mind wanders, my voice will go with you.

Now…begin to pay more attention to your body. You can begin to feel your feet touching the floor… And the back of your legs…notice the different parts of your back as it relaxes into the floor… See if you can visualise your relaxed body now as it is lying there getting more and more relaxed. *(Continue to pace and lead through the body for as long as you think it necessary, using a mixture of the hearing, seeing and feeling words.)*

And now you can start to watch and listen to your breath… just breathe in your normal relaxed way…there is no need to slow down the out-breath. Just observe the breathing… Start to pay special attention to your out-breath now…as this is the breath of relaxation… Each time you breathe out the body automatically relaxes and lets go. *(Stay with this as long as you need to.)*

Now to help you to relax even deeper, even further, I am going to count down from ten to one…and with each count you can relax even further, even deeper. With each count down you can relax ten times more.

Ten…let go, nine…eight…relax even deeper *(and so on – count down to one)* and…now, one, completely relaxed. Mentally and physically relaxed.

I would like you now to think of a place where you know you are comfortable, a place that is special to you. Just imagine that you can visit this place now in your imagination. What does this place look like, and what does it feel like to be in this place? I would like you to imagine that you are there now in this special place and that you are looking around you and seeing the things that you see. Look at the colours and shades. And what do you look like in this special place? And as you are looking around you now… how do you feel? Really enjoy this feeling, as it is part of you. You might get feelings in your body and really treasure those feelings of wellbeing and comfort. Are there any sounds associated with this place? And if there are, just hear them now. *(This is the time when you can add some suggestions of your objectives for the class. It could be general wellbeing, health, optimism, etc.)* Now...in a few moments' time I am going to count back from one to ten and by the time I reach eight you will start to move your body and by the time I count ten, you will be back with me in the present, fully aware and awake. You will come out of this deep state of relaxation with a feeling of wellbeing and a sense of oneness that will stay with you. You have learned that you can be relaxed at any time you wish. All you need to do is to remember how you feel now, see the pictures you see now and be aware of the sounds. This will bring back to you the sense of wellbeing that you are experiencing now. So now I am going to count one, two, three, four, five, six, seven, eight – start to move your body – nine, ten. Wide awake now. *(Bring them back to sitting in your own time.)*

To finish: magic words! 'That's right' and 'Now'

Milton Erickson, a respected psychiatrist and hypnotherapist, was one of the therapists Bandler and Grinder originally modelled. He was a very interesting man and quite a few NLP beliefs originated with him, such as: 'We have all the resources we need already within ourselves.' He had the habit of saying, 'That's right,' while he listened to his clients. The client's unconscious mind would feel reassured and resourced.

On one of my residential yoga retreats, a yoga student explained that she could not bend forward. This was, of course, a massive generalisation, as she actually bent forward many times a day. I invited her to sit on the stage with me and asked her to do *Paschimottanasana* (Sitting Forward Bend). She did and her fingertips reached just below her knees. I sat down next to her, matching her body and her breathing.

Each time she either moved, twitched and/or breathed out, I would say to her softly, 'That's right.' After a minute or so, she ended up touching her feet easily and by the end of the week she totally relaxed forward into the posture. It was a belief-change that made this possible. I did nothing proactive to make her change her mind that her body could do this movement. I have done this many times since, and every single time the student has felt there was the possibility that they could do more. Now I randomly say, 'That's right,' while I am teaching a whole class!

Ian McDermott, who was my main trainer at International Teaching Seminars (ITS), would call this 'relentless encouragement'.

When Milton Erickson worked with patients, he often just told them stories. Of course, his use of language was extremely effective and powerful and the stories would be metaphors, so the patients' healing and positive change would begin as they listened. Their unconscious attention was drawn to the stories in a number of ways, but especially through the word 'now'.

When I have something extremely relevant to say to the class or my clients that I really want them to hear and absorb, I always say: 'Now...' You will notice the word repeated many times in my relaxation script.

Just remember when you were young and someone wanted you to listen. Did they not say something like, 'And now I am going to tell you a story'?

If you have something really important to say to your classes, start the sentence with 'Now...'

And if it is beneficial for them to do something as well as they can, also start the instructions with 'Now...'

Now...that's right. Have fun playing with NLP!

— 7 —

Supporting Students with Injuries

Andrew McGonigle

As yoga becomes more and more popular each year and classes become busier, the likelihood of a student presenting to class with an injury increases. Many healthcare professionals are now recognising the potential benefits of yoga and are referring their clients in order to support injury rehabilitation. This puts a greater demand on the yoga teacher and adds to the challenge of teaching yoga safely. Busy classes with high turnovers, language barriers and students arriving late to class only add to this challenge.

This chapter aims to give you, the teacher, the knowledge and confidence you need to be able to approach, advise, support and empower students with common injuries that present to a yoga class.

I have not referenced scientific papers throughout this chapter because, first, there has not been as much research carried out on these topics as you might imagine and, second, I am not aiming to provide you with prescriptions that can be used to treat an injured student, because this goes beyond your role as a yoga teacher.

Why do we ask about injuries at the start of a class?

Let's start by discussing why it might be important to ask about injuries at the start of the class. As a teacher, we are there to guide a student or group of students safely through a practice that allows the student to develop awareness and explore their comfort zones without feeling pain or discomfort. Unless we are aware of their starting point, it is very difficult to engage in this process. By gathering basic information about where a student is at in their physical health on that day, we can begin a dialogue with them that helps to support and empower them. I strongly dislike being called a yoga *instructor*. I am not there to read a script and tell people what to do or what to feel. I am there to *teach*. One of my goals is to create an environment that encourages the student to compassionately learn about their body and become aware of their mind–body connection, their strengths and their limitations. By gaining an understanding of the challenges the student might be facing, we can offer advice and modifications that can allow the student to feel included while preventing them from precipitating any further injury.

If we are fortunate enough to teach in spaces that allow us access to yoga props, we can use blankets, belts, blocks, bricks and bolsters to support the students physically. Most of us are not trained yoga therapists or healthcare professionals. We are not qualified or insured to diagnose or treat students. Exploring why we ask about injuries can be a helpful and humbling reminder that we should try not to rise above our station as a yoga teacher. Remember that it is okay to say both 'I don't know,' and 'I don't feel that it is appropriate for you to take part in the class today.' This will often help build the trust between you as a teacher and the student. You might want to point the student in the direction of an experienced Pilates teacher, pre- or post-natal yoga teacher, physiotherapist or osteopath, particularly if you are encouraging them not to join the class. Finally, remember that it might also be a requirement of the studio or gym that you are teaching in and your insurance provider to ask students about injuries.

This brings us neatly on to the question: With whom does the responsibility lay when you are teaching an injured student?

The simple answer is that it is the responsibility of both the student and you as the teacher. The more complex answer is that responsibility lies with both parties, but it is your responsibility as a teacher to hold a space that allows an effective interaction to take place between yourself and the student, and it is the student's responsibility to take on-board your advice. Don't assume that students will necessarily know that it is important to tell you about a significant injury unless you ask. And don't assume that a student will listen to your advice after you have taken the time and effort to try to help them.

Case study

I was setting up to teach a busy open-level, hot yoga class and I interacted with a male student in his 40s who had been diagnosed with a herniated lumbar disc. I gave him the advice that I felt was appropriate for him and he confirmed that he understood. The class started and when we reached a specific *āsana* that I had given him a modification for, I noticed that he wasn't adhering to the advice that I had given him. I then engaged with him again and reiterated the advice. This happened a second time during the sequence and again I tried to intervene. When it happened the third time, I decided not to intervene directly but give more general guidance to the group regarding the *āsana* and what to do if one was experiencing feedback from their lower back. I had to shift the responsibility more towards the student himself, because by focusing the majority of my attention on him I was potentially impacting the group of students as a whole. At the end of the practice, I checked in with him to find out how his lower back had felt during the class.

Basic guidelines to adopt when approaching a student who has an injury

Let's take a moment to think about the most effective ways to ask a group of students about injuries. I would suggest avoiding creating an open forum where students discuss their injuries with you in front of the whole class. This could discourage shy students or those who may have a private matter that they would like to discuss with you. General questions like, 'Who has something that they feel they need to share with me?' can open a can of worms and have every hand in the class raising. I had a nightmare once where my class almost turned into a doctor's surgery, and by the time I had spoken to everyone we were halfway through the allotted time! I tend to say something like, 'If you are new to yoga or have something going on in your body that might be helpful to share with me, please raise your hand and I will come and have a brief chat with you.' This works well for me in the environment that I teach in, but you can adapt this to suit your own circumstances. I try to be the first person in the space and engage with students as they arrive. As more students arrive, I then address the whole group about five minutes prior to the start of the class and then speak to the last few students directly before the practice begins. Some teachers like to start the students in a supine position and invite them to raise a hand or place one hand on their abdomen if they need to talk to them about anything. You can give this a go and see how it works for you and your students.

As you approach a student who is sitting, it is helpful to come down to their level. Introduce yourself if they are new to you and ask their name. This might seem glaringly obvious, but it is worth taking a moment to consider. Start by clarifying what the actual injury is, for example do they know what 'I have a dodgy knee' actually means? Ask them how long they have had the injury. This raises the topic of acute versus sub-acute versus chronic injuries. If someone has sprained their ankle on the way to class, it won't be appropriate for them to practise. They will benefit from adopting the RICE treatment: rest, ice, compression and elevation. If the sprain happened a few days ago, it might be appropriate for them to join the class but take it easy, support themselves with props and modify a couple of specific *āsana*. If they had the injury two years ago, you might decide that they need very little advice and know exactly how to manage themselves. It is often helpful to ask the student how the injury limits them. This knowledge will help when deciding what modifications to suggest, which we will touch upon in a moment.

I have discussed this topic with many teachers, and this is the stage where we can get overwhelmed and feel insecure that we are not a walking encyclopaedia of medical conditions and how to manage them. Take a breath and feel secure in the knowledge that whatever the weird and wonderful condition or injury, we can approach the scenario in a logical way. It doesn't matter if the student is an orthopaedic surgeon who knows every detail about his knee injury or Joe Blogs with his vague 'dodgy' knee. Simply share with them the basic alignment principles that apply to the knee joint and let them know that they should back off if they feel any pain or discomfort in the joint. Did I hear a sigh of relief? It might be helpful to demonstrate what you mean to the student, without injuring yourself of course, and avoid using anatomical language that they might not understand. We will look at alignment principles in more detail later in the chapter.

The next step is to decide which of the *āsana* that you have planned to teach might have the tendency to make the particular injured joint vulnerable and offer appropriate modifications that can be adopted by the student. You can also offer the use of props here. If the venue that you teach in doesn't have props, it is a good idea for you to carry a few with you.

It is worth checking to make sure that the student understands what you have said and that they are following your guidance during the class. Use the end of the class as an opportunity to check in with the student after the practice to see how they feel and if they need any further guidance. Try your best to remember the student and their injury for when they come back to class and use this as a chance to clarify your advice if necessary. Often, offering general advice for when student is at home or at work can be really helpful. Tips on correcting bad posture or some exercises to help strengthen a weak area of the body can be very useful for the student.

Here is a checklist that you might find useful when engaging with an injured student.

- Come to their level, introduce yourself and ask their name.
- Clarify what the actual injury is, how long they have had it and how it limits them.
- Give general advice on alignment principles and backing off if they feel any discomfort.
- Offer modifications and/or use of props.
- Check to see that the student is following your guidance during class.
- Check in with the student after the class.
- Remember the student's issue for when they come back to class.
- Offer general, everyday advice for when the student is at home or at work.

Top tips for managing injured students when teaching large groups:

- Get to class early where possible.
- Set up the space, including props that might be useful.
- Ask about injuries as each student arrives, ask the group five minutes prior to the start of the class and ask again one minute before.
- If someone arrives late, try to approach them during the settling/warm up/contemplation.
- Engage with the students again at the end of class.

Common injuries

Here are some of the most common injuries that a student will present to class with:

- Shoulder: rotator cuff injury, shoulder impingement, dislocation, frozen shoulder.
- Knee: ligament damage, meniscal tears, arthritis, hypermobility.
- Lumbar spine: slipped/prolapsed/herniated/bulging discs, sciatica, general pain/tightness.
- Cervical spine: chronic neck tension/stiffness from incorrect head posture, slipped disc.
- Hamstring: attachment tear, strain.
- Sacroiliac (SI) joint: SI dysfunction.
- Elbow and wrist: hypermobility, repetitive strain injury (RSI), golfer's/tennis elbow, carpel tunnel syndrome.

A logical way to approach this huge topic is to briefly review the anatomy of the particular body part, focusing on why this area might be prone to injury in the first place. We can then look at general advice that could be given to a student, including basic alignment principles. It will be helpful to highlight some key *āsana* where particular attention needs to be made to that part of the body if injured and describe how these *āsana* could be modified or supported with props to accommodate such an injury. Finally, we can look at some simple techniques that can help to stabilise these areas of the body.

In the next section, we address how to apply this logical approach to the shoulder joint, knee joint and lumbar spine. The details here are by no means exhaustive and aim to serve as a guide to help you explore this topic with your students. There is also a detailed appendix to give you an overview of possible ways to approach the cervical spine, hamstrings, sacroiliac joint, elbow and wrist.

Exploring the shoulder joint

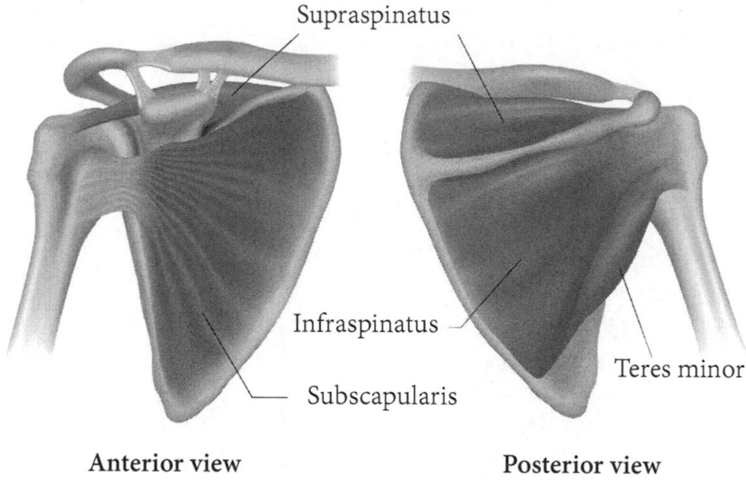

ROTATOR CUFF MUSCLES

Anatomy

The shoulder, or glenohumeral joint, is a ball-and-socket joint that involves the articulation between the head of the humerus and the glenoid fossa of the scapula. It is a shallow joint and has the greatest mobility of all joints. With this range of movement comes instability and a risk of dislocation. The glenoid labrum is a fibro-cartilaginous ring that provides additional depth and seals the joint. The joint is also sealed by a joint capsule and held in place by the glenohumeral ligaments. The capsule and ligaments are not very strong, but it is the role of the 'rotator cuff' muscles to stabilise the humeral head in the socket. Most people have no awareness of these muscles, and due to postural imbalances and inactivity they can become weak and often injured.

The infraspinatus lies below the spine of the scapula and inserts on the greater tuberosity of the humerus. It works alongside teres minor to produce external rotation of the shoulder joint. The supraspinatus lies above the spine of the scapula and also inserts on the greater tuberosity of the humerus. It initiates shoulder abduction and is the most frequent rotator cuff to become injured due to impingement. Impingement occurs when the tendon of the supraspinatus is compressed between the acromium of the scapula and the head of the humerus. In yoga this can occur when we are bearing weight on a shoulder joint that is internally rotated. External rotation of the joint draws the bony structures apart enough to free the supraspinatus tendon and prevent impingement.

Alignment

The key alignment principle relating to the shoulder joint is to have a degree of external rotation during flexion or extension, particularly when bearing weight on the joint. Note that hypermobile students may have the tendency to externally rotate too much, which is also a concern. In *āsana* like Plank Pose, the shoulders should be directly above the wrists to utilise the strength of the arm bones. Avoid hyperextending or locking the elbows, which can cause the shoulders to collapse. Correct scapula positioning is also key here. Preventing the lateral edge of the scapula from winging upwards during arm balances will take strain off the shoulder joint and keep the upper limb stable.

Āsana focus with suggested modifications

In Downward Dog, ensure that the arms are active while avoiding hyperextension of the elbows and that there is a degree of external rotation in the shoulder joint. Protraction and depression of the shoulder blades will also support this action. Those students with shoulder issues could try Downward Dog on their knees with their thighs vertical or use a chair to place their hands on. If you are lucky enough to teach in a studio with Iyengar ropes on the wall, you can teach Downward Dog with the hips supported by the ropes.

In Plank Pose, place a foam block between the hands to encourage activation of the arm muscles. Keep the shoulders externally rotated and offer the variation of knees on the ground for those who need the support.

In Shoulder Stand, place a thin blanket as support under the shoulders and ensure that the students realise that most weight will be going through the elbows and upper arms. Prevent the elbows from flaring to the sides, which will internally rotate the shoulder joints and potentially cause impingement.

How to stabilise the shoulder joints

A great exercise for engaging and building awareness of the rotator cuff muscles is to reach your arms forward with your palms facing and squeeze a block between your hands. Gently draw your arm bones back and down. Hold this for a few breaths and then repeat. Scapula press-ups can be used to build awareness of the stabilising action of protracting the shoulder blades. Start by facing a wall and placing your palms against the wall at shoulder height and shoulder width. Keeping your arms straight, isolate the retraction and protraction movements of your shoulder blades by drawing them towards each other and then drawing them apart and around the sides of your ribcage. You can then progress to doing this on all fours on the mat and eventually starting in a plank position. In arm balances where the palms are on the mat, energetically hugging the hands towards each other will engage the arm muscles and prevent elbow hyperextension.

Exploring the knee joint

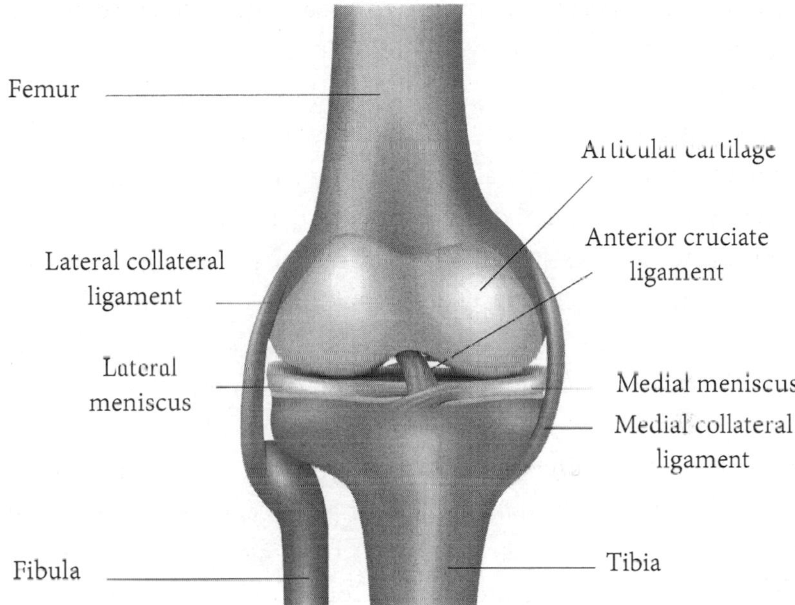

ANTERIOR VIEW OF THE RIGHT KNEE

Anatomy

The knee joint has the largest surface area of any joint in the body and is involved in both weight-bearing and movement. The knee is the relationship between the condyles of the femur and the condyles of the tibia and is primarily a hinge joint. It essentially only moves in two ways: into flexion and into extension. The knee can rotate a very small amount when flexed and can also hyperextend, but both of these movements should be avoided, particularly when weight-bearing on the knee joint.

Each knee has two fibro-cartilaginous C-shaped disc, called menisci, that are positioned medially and laterally. The function of the menisci is to aid the spreading of synovial fluid during movement, increase the weight-bearing surface and provide stability through their wedge shape. The menisci are prone to injury, particularly the posterior aspect of the medial meniscus, due to the bony structure. Injury can occur during compression, squatting or rotation. Since the menisci are cartilaginous, they do not have a direct blood supply and are very slow to heal.

There are two main sets of ligaments in the knee: the collateral ligaments (medial and lateral) and the cruciate ligaments (anterior and posterior). The medial and lateral collateral ligaments hold the knee joint in place and resist medial and lateral displacement respectively. Rotating the knee joint internally or externally will potentially strain these ligaments. They are exterior to the joint capsule, and while injury to these ligaments can be very painful, they are capable of healing on their own. The anterior and posterior cruciate ligaments resist anterior and posterior displacement respectively. The anterior cruciate also limits knee rotation. In an *āsana* like Chair Pose, *Utkatasana*, drawing the knees too far past the ankles will potentially strain the posterior cruciate ligament. Hyperextending or locking the knee can strain the anterior cruciate ligament. These ligaments are inside the joint capsule and do not have their own blood supply. It is therefore very difficult for these ligaments to heal independently.

Alignment

Our knees work hard every day and intelligent alignment is essential in order to build strength and stability. With our anatomy in mind, we want to avoid collapsing or compressing either side of the joint. We should aim to balance lateral and medial structures to align the knee cap, and in both flexed and extended positions keep both hamstrings and quadriceps active, hugging the joint together.

Tight hips can refer tension directly to the knee, particularly during hip rotation. Keeping the feet active by spreading the toes and everting/pronating the ankle joints will engage the muscles around the knee to protect it.

Here are some keys alignment cues to help protect the knee joints during an *āsana* practice.

- When bending the knee in standing positions, keep it in line with the mid-point of your ankle to avoid the knee rolling inwards or outwards.
- In lunge positions, keep the knee stacked above your ankle so that the shin bone (tibia) is vertical.
- Avoid hyperextending or locking the knee joint, particularly in standing poses.
- Activating your feet by spreading your toes will engage the muscles around your knee joint and protect it, particularly when releasing tight hips.
- Never press against the knee joint itself.
- The knee joints shouldn't feel painful or uncomfortable during the practice. If they do, back off from what you are doing.

Āsana focus with suggested modifications

In Pigeon Pose, keep the front foot active by spreading the toes and pressing into the ball of the big toe. If necessary, support the pelvis with a block so that the hips are level. Supine Pigeon is a really accessible alternative here and it can even be practised against a wall so that the upper body can relax.

In Chair Pose, squeeze a block between the thighs to keep the knees tracking over the ankles. You can also place a block between the feet to keep them parallel. Spread the toes to keep the inner arches of the feet engaged.

In Hero Pose, peel the calf muscle down but not out to prevent the knee from rotating. Support the seat with a block or, as an alternative *āsana*, try Saddle Pose with the big toes touching and knees wide.

Top tips for building knee stability

- Build the integrity of the inner arches of the feet by spreading and lifting the toes.
- Release tight hip muscles.
- Strengthen the gluteal muscles to better support the pelvis and hip joints.
- Become aware of locking the knees in everyday life.

Exploring the lumbar spine

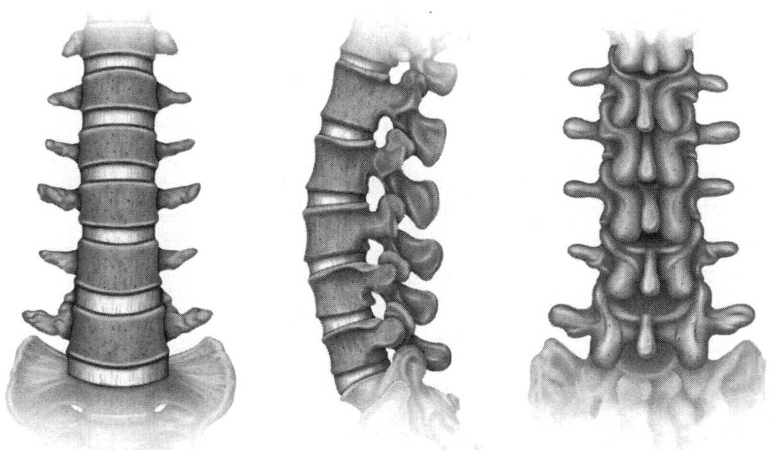

ANTERIOR, LATERAL AND POSTERIOR VIEW OF THE LUMBAR VERTEBRAE

Anatomy

The lumbar spine comprises five vertebrae that lie between the pelvis and the lower ribcage. It is concave posteriorly, giving a natural lumbar lordosis curve. This part of the spine supports much of our body weight and the vertebrae are large with thick intervertebral discs to compensate for this. The lumbar spine relies on a series of deep muscles for support. Due to lack of awareness of these muscles, lack of exercise and poor postural habits, these muscles are often weak.

The average range of movement in the lumbar spine is as follows: 60° flexion, 35° extension, 20° lateral flexion and 5° rotation. Therefore, while the lumbar spine is designed for backbending, forward folding and side bending, it is not designed for twisting movements.

Between adjacent vertebrae lie intervertebral discs that facilitate movement, as well as acting as shock absorbers and weight-bearers. The discs can't actually slip, but they can herniate, rupture or prolapse, putting pressure on the spinal cord and the nerves as they exit the spinal column. Risk factors for disc problems include sedentary lifestyle, obesity, weak core muscles, trauma, ageing and dehydration. Most pressure is exerted on the intervertebral discs during prolonged sitting and forward bending. The intervertebral discs have no internal blood supply and limited external blood supply and are therefore very slow to heal if damaged. Supported movement of the spine helps to move fluid in and out of the discs and keep them hydrated and healthy.

Alignment

Here are some tops tips for supporting your lower back during yoga.

- Listen to any feedback that your lower back is giving you during your yoga practice and back off if necessary. Remember that your practice should feel good in your body.

- Avoid rounding your lower back in forward folds. Try sitting on a block to raise your seat and lengthen your spine as you fold. Bend your knees slightly to release the hamstrings at the back of your pelvis and allow the pelvis to tilt forward.

- When setting yourself up for backbending, start by rolling your inner thighs back and then lower your tailbone down to lengthen your lower back.

- Engage your core muscles, which will act as a corset around your lower back supporting the vertebrae. Lengthening your spine along its axis will engage these muscles and you can actively draw your lower belly up and in for additional support.
- Avoid twisting in your lower back. Keep your hips square so that your spine and pelvis don't move in opposite directions. In seated twists, avoid pressing your outer arm into your outer knee, but press down to support your spine to lengthen.

Āsana focus with suggested modifications

In Camel Pose, lengthen the lower back by rolling the inner thighs back and rooting the tailbone. Avoid 'tucking' the tailbone, which can cause the gluteal muscles to grip. A block between the thighs can help to keep the legs active. Either keep the hands on the hips or place a bolster on top of the ankles to act as a support for the hands and encourage length through the thoracic spine. Bridge Pose is a useful alternative here.

In standing forward folds, either place the hands on the shins or thighs or on two blocks placed in front. Avoid reaching the arms forward as the body folds to reduce strain on the lower back. Encourage a soft bend to the knees allowing the spine to lengthen forward. Engaging the lower abdominal muscles will support the lower back. Avoid rounding through the spine by keeping the *Drishti* forward.

In Downward Dog, bend the knees deeply as the hips lift higher, allowing the lower back to lengthen. Tone the lower belly up and in. Pressing the hands into the mat will encourage further length in the spine.

How to stabilise the lower back

Prone backbends can be a great way to strengthen the lower back. Start in Baby Cobra, keeping the hands pressing down and back. Lengthen the sternum forward as the tailbone and feet reach back. Then gradually build to lifting the hands an inch off the mat.

Doing dedicated core work such as Pilates is a wonderful way to support your lower back. Invest in an exercise ball to improve your posture at home.

Releasing tight hamstring and psoas muscles can relieve pressure from the lower back. Developing appropriate gluteal muscle engagement can also start to address muscular imbalances across your pelvis.

Refer to the appendix for a summary of all major joints that are prone to injury and a review of the anatomy and relevant *āsana* that may be impacted. This is here to serve as a guide and the information is not exhaustive.

Suggested homework

Find a colleague, friend or family member who has an injury. Review the anatomy related to this injury. Describe the advice that you would offer this person if they came to one of your yoga classes. Which *āsana* would they need to be particularly mindful of and how could these *āsana* be modified or supported with props?

Appendix

How to support injured students: overview

Body part	Common injuries	Anatomy review	Alignment advice	Asana focus	Modifications	How to stabilise
Shoulder	Rotator cuff tear, impingement, dislocation, frozen shoulder	Most mobile joint Weak capsule and ligaments Reliant on rotator cuff muscles for stability Bad posture leads to muscular imbalances	Engaging the head of the humerus into the socket Avoiding extreme external or internal rotation when weight-bearing Stabilising the shoulder blades Avoiding elbow hyperextension	Any weight-bearing pose, Downward Dog, Plank, Caturaṅga, Crow, Shoulder Stand	Downward Dog with knees on the ground and thighs vertical Downward Dog with a chair or using Iyengar ropes Plank on forearms	Rotator cuff exercise: straighten arms in front, squeeze a block between hands, draw heads of humerus back and down Explore scapula press-ups against wall to develop scapula stabilisation Avoid hyperextending the elbows

Knee	Cruciate/ collateral ligament issues, meniscal tears, arthritis, hypermobility	Large weight-bearing joint, relies on strong ligaments for stability Tight hips and flat feet arches have a huge impact	When weight-bearing the knee must be directly above the ankle and in line with the ankle in the sagittal plane Activate feet and ankles and release tight hips Micro-bend knee	Warriors, Sukhasana, Padmasana, Pigeon, Malasana, Utkatasana, Bow Pose	Supine Pigeon as a hip opener variation Block between thighs in Utkatasana Support under knees in Sukhasana	Build the inner arches of the feet Use toe spreaders Supine Padangusthasana in three stages to engage the leg muscles Supine Pigeon to release tight outer hips Postural advice to avoid locking the knees
Neck	Arthritis, chronic neck tension, slipped disc	No intervertebral disc between C1 and C2 Five kg head! Largest range of movement in the spine	No weight-bearing No 'crunching' back of the neck Only extend neck if it feels good Correct head position: ears in line with shoulders	Shoulder Stand, Head Stand, Tāḍāsana, Trikoṇāsana, Ustrasana	Shoulder Stand with props Option for legs up the wall Avoid extending or rotating	Develop correct head posture Release tension with massage Supportive pillow Neck stretches

Body part	Common injuries	Anatomy review	Alignment advice	Asana focus	Modifications	How to stabilise
Lumbar	Slipped/ prolapsed/ herniated/bulging discs, sciatica	Weight-bearing, large range of movement but little rotation Relies on muscular stabilisation Impacted by the pelvic tilt	Avoid rounding Lengthen the lower back by rolling the inner thighs back and rooting the tailbone Treat backbends more as chest openers Back off if any pain Avoid using the arms as levers	Ustrasana, Dancer's Pose, Utkatasana, Bow Pose	Squeeze a block between the thighs Bend knees in forward fold Avoid rolling up from a forward fold.	Baby Cobra Pose and similar prone backbends Core work Correct standing and sitting posture Releasing hamstrings and psoas
Hamstring	Attachment tear	Polyarticular, tightens with running/sport Often over used because of weak glutes, can compensate for tight lower back	Avoid hyperextension Bend knees! Gentle stretching without pain Mindful movement Patience!	Paschimottanasana, Janu Shirasana, Uttanasana	Bend knees! Sit on a blanket Use strap for support Gently contract the muscles while stretching them	Engaging the glutes to take pressure off the hamstrings Addressing postural imbalances Gentle stretching in Supine Padangusthasana

SI joint	SI joint dysfunction	Junction between lower limbs and spine Too little or too much movement Reliant on ligaments for stability Only the piriformis is directly attached	Avoid forcing the hip bone and the thigh bone in opposite directions Keep the hips square in forward folds Move the pelvis as one integrated unit	Trikoṇāsana, Janu Shirasana, Utthita Hasta Padangusthasana, Garbha Pindasana, Warrior Two	Avoid asymmetrical poses Avoid fixing the pelvis in twists Use a foam block to keep the pelvis level in forward folds Ensure symmetry in restorative postures	Develop a 'snugness' at the back of the pelvis Release tight piriformis and hamstrings Inner core work to provide stability Engage adductors Address psoas and quadratus lumborum (QL) imbalances Refer to a medical professional

Body part	Common injuries	Anatomy review	Alignment advice	Asana focus	Modifications	How to stabilise
Elbow/ wrist	Hypermobility, RSI, golfer's/ tennis elbow, carpel tunnel syndrome	Hinge joint, some people can lock the elbow and some can't We flex our wrists a lot during the day Tight neck and shoulders can lead to elbow and wrist issues	Spread the fingers wide with the index fingers parallel Wrist directly under shoulders when weight-bearing Avoid locking the elbow: micro-bend the elbow, roll the elbow crease in the direction of the thumb and then draw the hands towards one another, straightening the arms	Downward Dog, Cat Cow, Plank, *Prasārita Padottanāsana* C	Fists in Cat Cow to support wrists Downward Dog with knees on mat and thighs vertical Downward Dog with Iyengar ropes Plank on forearms	Wrist extension can be helpful as well as working to loosen up tight trapezius and neck muscles

This list is not exhaustive and is here as a guide only.

— 8 —

Yoga Adjustments

Melanie Cooper

What are adjustments?

When teaching yoga there are several ways to explain poses to students:

- verbal descriptions
- visual demonstration
- hands-on guidance.

Adjustments are hands-on guidance that use physical touch to help your teaching. Adjustments are not something that the teacher 'does' to the student; they are a dialogue – something you do together. The start of the dialogue has to be permission: does the student want to be touched in this pose and on this day? It's of paramount importance to find a way to check with your students if they want to be adjusted and even more important to make sure you explicitly give them an easy way to say no to an adjustment. There will be more on this later in the chapter. So, an adjustment is a dialogue: you, as the teacher, are making a suggestion with your touch and the student is choosing whether that suggestion feels good to them. The beauty of this is that it can be done in silence, without breaking the flow of the practice. It can be done with connection and nurturing. It can be done gently with love and care.

Why adjust?

Before going into the nuts and bolts of adjusting, it's important to look at why we adjust. Why not let students find their own alignment and depth in a pose? With recent increased awareness of injuries caused by yoga practice and adjustments, trauma sensitivity in those who have been hurt and abused in the past and the many sexual scandals hitting the yoga world – why still adjust?

These are all valid questions and valid reasons for not touching someone in a yoga class. Many yoga teachers decide they don't want to risk injuring someone in an adjustment or inadvertently invading someone's space, particularly male teachers. I'd recommend having a long, hard and honest think about adjustments – what are your reasons for adjusting? What do you want to 'achieve' by adjusting? What do you want to give the student?

Having said that, personally I find adjustments one of the best parts of teaching and, having taught for 20 years, it's the thing that keeps me interested, engaged and inspired as a teacher. I think that human touch is natural and healing. There are many studies showing that hospital patients who are touched heal quicker than those who are not touched. In the context of yoga poses, adjustments can be used in many ways – there is far more to adjustments than taking someone deeper into a pose, although sometimes this is appropriate too.

Adjustments don't have to be strong and deep; sometimes a small correction can transform a student's practice. Let's look at some detail of why we adjust.

To give foundation

In standing poses, this normally means holding the outside of the hips and firmly pressing in towards the centre line of the body.

In sitting poses, it normally means pressing the sit bones back and down towards the floor.

Sometimes, pressing the student's foot into the floor is the most helpful.

When the foundation is secure and stable, it's possible for the student to explore the posture more freely; for example in a seated twist, if you place your foot over the student's foot and gently press down, it might enable them to lift up more through the spine, and this may enable them to go more deeply into the twist. If you place your foot gently over the student's supporting foot in a standing balance, it often enables them to lift up more into the pose and focus on alignment instead of just struggling to find and hold the balance.

To give stability

For some people, balancing in poses is a real challenge and while it is good for people to work on their balance and find more stability, it can be very frustrating to be falling out of poses all the time. People who often find balancing a challenge if they:

- are very tall, with a high centre of balance
- have fallen arches in the feet
- are pregnant, as the centre of balance has changed
- have hypermobility syndrome, meaning they can have problems with proprioception, which can also make it hard to balance.

An adjustment that gives the lightest touch to reiterate the foundation can enable the student to work on a pose without falling completely, which can be very helpful and avoid a lot of frustration.

To connect to core strength

Many students have a habit of overarching the lower back. In this position, the abdominal muscles are held too long. In order to function optimally, a muscle needs to be held at just the right length (the Goldilocks Principle); if the muscle is held too short or too long, it can't function effectively. If you can guide the body back to a position where the lower back is in its functional position (normally neutral curves in the spine), this will help a student to connect to their core strength. This overarching of the lower back can often be seen in Warrior One (*Vīrabhadrāsana I*), in the preparation and movement into standing forward bends and in Chair Pose (*Utkatasana*).

To show which way to go

For some students, especially those who are hypermobile, knowing which way to go in a pose is one of their main challenges. Going the 'wrong way' can mean missing the benefits of the pose and sometimes creating shortening or tension in the body. For example, Reverse Triangle (*Parivrtta Trikoṇāsana*) is a pose where students often go the 'wrong way'. As a student works towards the flexibility to place the hand on the floor, the torso is moving down and towards the mid-line of the pose. It's really common for students to then carry on going past the mid-line and end up with the torso in a scrunched up 'C' shape. An adjustment (often in conjunction with a verbal explanation) can place the student back in a place of length and openness. Another common example is the shoulders in Downward Dog (*Adho Mukha Svanasana*). Often, students start with the shoulders stiff and the arm slightly bent. They start to stretch, bringing the chest towards the knees, but there comes a certain point when this journey needs to stop otherwise the shoulders will end up internally rotated and hunched up towards the ears. An adjustment can draw the shoulders back to an open, relaxed position.

To give alignment

While it is important to acknowledge there is no such thing as one correct alignment that will suit all bodies, and we are not trying to squash different body types into a 'perfect *āsana*' mould, I think it is true to say that there are certain common misalignments that can often cause wear and tear to joints, tension to muscles and possibly injury.

Often, people have a habit of either overarching their lower back or tucking their tail bone under and flattening the lower back. Both of these habits can cause wear and tear on the vertebrae and spinal disks and can cause the abdominal muscles to become weak and lax in the first case and weak and tight in the second. An adjustment can help to keep the neutral curves in the spine and help a student feel where neutral is.

Shoulders are another area that often come out of alignment, creeping forwards and up towards the ears, possibly causing tension and stress to the body, especially the upper trapezius muscle and causing the muscles of the upper back, such as the rhomboid, to become weak. An adjustment can help a student to find openness and balance in the shoulder area.

To connect to the breath

Often, students find staying connected to a slow, deep, powerful breath a challenge. It's definitely the case that if a student's breath is shallow and fast, a strong, deep adjustment is not a good idea and could cause injury. This is because when the breath is fast and shallow, it's a signal to the nervous system to get ready for action, and tensing muscles is part of this process. To connect a student to their breath you can place your hands on the ribcage, breathe slow and deep yourself, indicate gently with the hands how the body can move with the breath and also maybe give a verbal suggestion to 'slow down the breath'.

To connect and nurture

Human touch is healing and nurturing; it creates connection and resonance between the teacher and student. As a teacher, sometimes it's only when you touch a student in an adjustment that you get certain information, such as whether they tense and pushing in the pose or whether they are breathing right.

How to make adjustments safe

Permission

The first and most important rule of when not to adjust is when the student has said 'No'. 'No' means 'No'! You absolutely must respect it and not try to persuade a student if they have said they don't want to be adjusted.

It is best practice to give students clear permission to say 'no' to an adjustment or to ask you to be softer during an adjustment.

It is important to tell students explicitly that adjustments shouldn't hurt and that if at any time an adjustment feels as if it is too much, they can say, 'That's enough.' Also, if on a particular day they don't feel like receiving adjustments, it's fine to say 'Not today.'

There are certain adjustments that are often intense to receive – for example, binding in *Marichyasana* D (Half Lotus Bound Twist), *Supta Kurmasana* (Sleeping Tortoise) and *Kapotasana* (Pigeon Pose). For intense poses, ask permission every time. 'Is it okay today?' or just 'Okay?' are enough.

Explain about the pain

Many students come to yoga thinking it should hurt, and the more it hurts the harder they are working and the more benefits they will get. It's important to persuade people that this is not the case. If the body is stretched too hard, the nervous system steps in to tighten the muscles to protect them. Soft and gentle really is more effective. Explain to students that adjustments should not hurt. They should feel good. They should enable and support the student to find their best version of the pose ('best' meaning most beneficial for the body and mind).

Beginners

With beginners, it's best practice to use small corrections, gentle guidance and never strong adjustments. It takes most beginners a while just to get used to 'making the shape' of the *āsana*. Anything beyond that, such as knowing how to work the pose, knowing how to play the edge and knowing which way to go within the pose, usually come later. In order for a student to 'receive' an adjustment with awareness of when to say 'no' – knowing the difference between a good sensation and the sensation of potential injury – they normally need a fair bit of experience and time to develop self-awareness. With beginners, small corrections can be very helpful. Beginners often don't 'get it' through a verbal explanation or demonstration, so using gentle, hands-on suggestions can be far more effective and useful to a beginner. It also creates a bond and connection between the student and teacher

Hypermobility

Hypermobility is a syndrome where the ligaments around a joint are more lax or loose than 'normal'. This comes with several challenges. You can recognise someone with hypermobility, as they often have more than 'normal' range of motion in their elbow and knees and often have overarching (hyper-lordosis) in their lower back. This means that if they go right to the end of their range of motion, they are pushing into ligaments and are possibly destabilising their joints. The best strategy for them in their yoga practice is to focus on drawing in, stabilising and connecting to their core strength. Any adjustments given to a student with hypermobility will be most helpful to the student if they do not 'stretch them further into the pose', but instead connect them to their foundation or core strength.

Students with hypermobility often also have problems with sacraliliac (SI) joint pain and collapsed arches in the feet. They also often don't 'feel' the stretch. This means that common yoga cues such as 'fold forward until you feel a gentle stretch' can have them stretching and stretching and thinking 'Where is this stretch supposed to be?' If you have a hypermobile student in your class, make sure to add in alternative cues, such as 'If you are hypermobile, press the sit bones back and down, keep drawing the navel in and up and don't worry about how far forwards you go.'

Hypermobile students often have difficulty knowing where their body is in space (proprioception). Often, you can give a cue such as 'arms at shoulder height' and their arms are anywhere but shoulder height. A gentle correction here will be helpful. Adjustments that give the information of where a student is in space can generally be helpful for hypermobile students.

Injuries

I hope it's fairly obvious that it is a very bad idea to do an adjustment on a body part that is already injured. But maybe it's not always obvious that if someone is injured in their shoulder, for example, there are probably lines of tension running all round the body and care should be taken with the hips even though they aren't close to the site of the injury. This is because when an injury happens, the body unconsciously and naturally tightens up muscles around that area to try to keep it still and protect it while it heals. Muscles don't exist in isolation in the body – our current model of anatomy suggests they exist as interconnected chains of muscles. This means that an injury and general tightness in the muscles around it can cause tightness elsewhere; for example, an injury in the neck can cause tightness in the lower back. If a student has an injury, completely avoid the injured area and go very gently and slowly even while adjusting them elsewhere in the body.

Pregnancy

There are a few aspects of pregnancy that mean it is best not to give adjustments. The first is the hormone relaxin. This hormone starts to be released at some point during pregnancy, often in the first trimester, so it's best to make allowances right from the beginning. It also stays after the birth, so it's important to be careful after the birth as well. Its purpose is to soften the joints for birth, but it softens all the joints and not just the ones necessary for birth. The best advice to a pregnant student is to go to 80 per cent of their 'edge'. That means don't push until the stretch is felt: stay just in the sensation-free range. This will avoid joints being overstretched and injured.

In pregnancy, no pressure should be put on the abdomen.

The best rule to follow is no adjustments for pregnant students, but balances are an exception. During pregnancy, the centre of balance changes, which means that a pregnant student can be a bit wobbly in balances. It's best not to have pregnant ladies falling over in yoga classes, so I normally give gentle support so they keep strengthening the legs but are not at risk of falling over.

Another exception is SI joint pain. If a pregnant student experiences pain at the SI joint, it's important that they don't push into it and try to 'stretch it out'. The best advice is to draw back, stabilise and work on strengthening the muscles in the hips, especially the gluteus group (muscles in the buttocks). In terms of adjustments, you can help to stabilise the hips so the pregnant student doesn't overuse and overstretch the SI joint. You can do this by holding the outside of the hips and pressing into the centre line.

The student can strengthen the gluteus muscles by doing 'Superman' Pose, i.e. being on all fours and lifting up the legs, one at a time, straight behind them. This also strengthens the abdominal muscles in a healthy way for pregnant students.

Pushers

Some students come to their yoga practice with an attitude of pushing and pulling themselves into the pose, come what may. They will pull their feet to get further into a forward bend, creating tension in their shoulders and putting their muscles and joints at risk of serious injury. They will push with their head into backbends and twists. If an adjustment is given, it can make the pose even more stressful for the body. It is up to the yoga teacher to encourage these students to back off and go more gently. The nervous system has a mechanism called the 'stretch reflex' that monitors if a muscle is being stretched too hard or too fast. If this is the case, it sends a message to the muscle to tense up for protection. This means that a soft and gentle stretch will actually be safer and more effective for the body. Any adjustment given in this case needs to encourage softening or backing off, for example grounding the sit bones in a forward bend.

Breath

If a student has short, shallow breath, this will send a signal to the nervous system to tense the body up ready for action – part of the flight or fight mechanism. If a student's breath isn't slow and deep, their muscles are probably tense, so it's best not to give an adjustment.

Wide-legged forward bends

One of the muscles on the inside of the thigh (the adductor magnus) is vulnerable in wide-legged forward bends. This is because it attaches to the sit bone (ischial tuberosity), which means it acts as an adductor and as a hamstring (the muscles on the back of the thighs). So in a wide-legged forward bend, it is under a double stretch acting as both an adductor (when the legs are taken wide apart) and a hamstring (in the forward fold). This means that it can be easily pulled to the end of its range and injured. The only adjustment to give that is safe is to reiterate the foundation and give grounding (not to take a student deeper).

Gentle in Prasārita Padottanāsana C!

Prasārita Padottanāsana C is a wide-legged, standing, forward fold where the hands are interlaced behind the back and the arms are taken up and over the head and down towards the floor. In this pose, the joint at the front of the shoulder (the acromioclavicular (AC) joint) is very vulnerable. A long lever can exert a big force, so a small amount of pressure on the arms (in this case long levers) can translate to a large force on the other end (the shoulders and the AC joint). If you are adjusting this pose, fingertip pressure at the hands is enough to give a strong adjustment at the shoulders.

Knots of tension

If a knot of tension has formed in a muscle (e.g. around an old injury), the knot itself is unlikely to respond to stretching. This means that the muscle fibre around it is likely to tear. Muscle knots are best dealt with through massage by a professional.

Not on a joint

Joints are the most vulnerable places in the body, so always avoid putting pressure on a joint. This particularly applies to the spine and the knees, especially when the knee is in lotus.

Potential pitfalls

Giving diagnoses and trying to fix people

When using hands-on adjustments, there are many potential pitfalls. First, it is important to remember that we are not diagnosing physical problems, we are not physical therapists and we are not fixing people. Students will want you to help them with physical problems, and you want to help! But, as a yoga teacher, you are not a physical therapist and not qualified or trained to work on this level. Physiotherapists and other body workers spend years studying to do this. You can't learn it on a 200-hour teacher training. Maybe with study and experience you can make an educated guess, but it's best practice to have a properly qualified body worker you know and trust, who understands yoga, to whom you can refer people for proper diagnosis and to learn how to adapt their yoga practice.

Trauma sensitivity

Another potential pitfall is students who have past or present trauma and feel uncomfortable or invaded by physical touch. You need to have a way of allowing these people to say 'no' to touch in an easy and non-judgemental way. You could give all students a card saying 'yes' on one side and 'no' on the other. They could leave this card by their mat so you can see who wants to be adjusted on any given day. Or you could give all new students a form to fill in that asks if they want to receive adjustments. Or you could ask verbally, 'Do you want to be adjusted?' and emphasise clearly that, 'It's fine to say no.' Adjustment cards don't have to be expensive or complicated: you could use a normal pack of playing cards and face up means 'yes' and face down means 'no'.

There are more and more Trauma Sensitive yoga courses being offered. It's definitely worth learning how to adapt your teaching so it feels welcoming and safe for everyone.

Let's do it!

General guidelines

START AT THE BEGINNING

If you are going to do an adjustment, first wait for the student to get into the pose. Don't jump on them as they're just getting in. Then start the adjustment at the start of the pose. It can be annoying for someone to come and give an adjustment just as you are coming out at the end of the pose.

STAY FOR THE WHOLE POSE

Don't just give a little push or shove and then go off and do something else; stay for the whole pose. Even if the body doesn't seem to be responding to your adjustment, stay, keep contact, breathe and soften and work on yourself. This will somehow transmit to the student; they will feel it through your hands. You could check your own alignment – could you soften your shoulders down? Are you using your core strength? Check your own breathing – could your breath be slower or deeper? Could it be more powerful?

DO BOTH SIDES

If the pose has two sides, then do both. Being adjusted on only one side can leave a student feeling wonky.

INCLUDE EVERYONE

There will be some students you are naturally attracted to more than others, but it's important that you don't just give all your attention to a few students. Share your attention out equally, include everyone and don't have favourites.

HOW TO USE THE TOUCH

Use the whole hand. If you use just a part of the hand – the heel of the hand or the fingertips, for example – the student is likely to feel as if they're being poked in an unpleasant way. It is best to use the whole hand and to keep the hand relaxed; this will give the student the best experience.

Touch exercises

How hard to adjust

There is a way of touching that is firm and confident: not too hard or too soft. Too hard will feel rough and harsh for the student and too soft will feel annoying and maybe creepy. To practise this, find someone to receive your touch and give good, honest feedback. Stand behind them and place your hands on their shoulders. First do it too soft, then do it hard and then find the middle ground clear and confident. Check with them that you've got it right.

Sensitivity

To work on your sensitivity, have them lie down. Sit at their head and hold their head in your hands with your hands resting on the ground. Then just tune in. See what you can feel, such as the texture and feel of their skin, the bones and muscles under the skin and the pulse of the cerebrospinal fluid. Stay like this for a few minutes and then slowly release your contact. Let them take some time to come back to sitting and ask them to feed back. Often, this very simple touch and tuning in is very powerful. It is profoundly nurturing, relaxing and healing. This is what you can give through adjustments: this connection and love.

DON'T GO UNDER CLOTHES

You might not even notice if your finger slips under the edge of someone's t-shirt, but to the student it can feel creepy and invasive, so make sure you stay on top of clothing.

RED-LIGHT AND AMBER-LIGHT AREAS

There are some areas of the body that you absolutely should never touch – the groin, genitals and chest. These are red-light areas – don't touch! Then there are sensitive areas – called amber-light areas – that are close to the red-light areas. It can be okay to touch these areas, but care must be taken. For example, it can be okay to touch the sides of the hips around the greater trochanter, but not to touch buttocks themselves. It can be okay to touch the shoulder close to the chest, but not the chest itself. It is sometimes acceptable to touch these areas, but it's important to be very clear in your intention and make sure that as you are making contact you don't fumble and move your hand around: just make one clear, firm connection. The same applies when you are releasing contact: remove your hand completely in one movement. If you feel uncomfortable and are thinking 'I wonder if the student thinks I'm being creepy and inappropriate,' then it's highly likely that the student *will* feel uncomfortable and unhappy about the adjustment.

I would only use adjustments involving amber-light areas with students I know well and I know are comfortable with touch. If in doubt, don't do the adjustment.

I include these 'amber-light adjustments' because they can give fantastic results, but you do have to be sensitive and aware and judge when they are appropriate and when they are not.

Protect yourself when adjusting

It is not uncommon for yoga teachers to injure themselves when doing adjustments. Following some simple guidelines can reduce this risk.

- Always stay connected to your core strength.
- If an adjustment involves bending forwards and taking weight, be especially careful to bend your knees, keep the back straight and engage the abdominals.
- Remember, just as a student can say 'no' to an adjustment, you can too. If a student is asking you to do something you don't feel confident with, or don't feel strong enough to do, say 'no'.
- Only do adjustments on poses you do yourself. You need to have the experience of what that pose feels like in order to fully understand how the pose works.
- Keep your shoulders back and down and engage the strong back muscles.
- Whenever possible, use the strength in the legs rather than the arms.
- Stay focused on what you are doing, not what you are going to do next.

Your foundation

The first part of any adjustment is to get your own foundation balanced and relaxed. If you aren't comfortable in your foundation, you could overbalance and push too hard in the adjustment or the adjustment could just turn out unstable and uncomfortable for the student. If you are unbalanced and tense at all, you will communicate that through your hands. Consciously or unconsciously, the student will feel it and be aware of it.

Use your body weight and don't push

If you do all of your adjustment pushing with your strength, you will tire yourself out by the end of teaching and the adjustment will feel harsher to the student. Place your whole hand on the body and then sink in gently with your body weight. It's easier for you and feels nicer to the student.

Adjust with the breath and breathe with student

The body naturally relaxes and releases with the exhalation. For forward bends and twists, always do any sinking deeper on the exhalation; for backbends, the lift and work into the pose is on the inhalation.

If you breathe with the student, it creates a connection and reminds them to keep breathing slowly and deeply.

Focus on yourself

Whatever you are feeling will be communicated to the student. After 20 years of giving adjustments pretty much on a daily basis, it's one of the main things I've learned. I set my foundation, connect to my core strength, place my hands on the body, think of what I'm hoping to give to the student and then I focus on myself: I keep my own shoulders relaxed, stay connected to my core strength, lengthen or twist my spine and soften and ease myself forwards. How the student feels it and comes with you is like magic. It feels amazing, beautiful, soft and healing.

Feel your own body

When you fully connect with someone else and make physical contact, you can actually feel in your own body what's going on in the student's body. So, if you feel the student isn't responding to the adjustment, feel what's happening in your body and see if that can inform what you do next.

Also, just be a witness. Feel the sensations in your hands as you touch their body – can you feel the layers of the skin, the bones and the muscles? Really tune in and feel as much as you can. This has the effect of allowing the body to 'tell its story'. It sometimes helps to tell someone about something that's bothering you: it can help to have someone really listen, even if they don't have the solution. The same is true of the body: listen and feel what's happening in the student's body and that can be very profound and healing. Try the sensitivity touch exercise on page 142 to really feel for yourself how powerful a simple touch can be.

How hard to adjust

Initially, one of the most difficult aspects of adjusting is developing the sensitivity to judge how deep to go. But, like most things, doing great, sensitive adjustments is a mixture of technique and practice. The general guidelines are to: make contact with the student and then tune into their breath; as they exhale, gently sink in with your body weight, keeping your hands and arm as relaxed as possible; when you feel resistance, stop and give a little space. Wait to see if the resistance softens and you can go deeper; if not, just stay there and breathe with the student. While you're adjusting, it's important to look for signs that the student has reached their limit. Signs to back off are if the:

- breathing becomes shallow or quicker
- body starts to shake
- student tenses their face
- student pushes back against your hand.

Finally, if in doubt, ask, 'Is that too much?' or, 'Could it be more gentle?'

Less is more

In the past, many teachers (myself included) were quite strong and hard in giving adjustments. This often came from a place of wanting to help the student achieve all they were capable of, but often it created an attitude of striving and making injuries more likely.

As time has gone by and I have got older and softer, I have become more and more gentle in my adjustments. I have come to focus far more on breathing with the student and on relaxing myself as much as I can. It seems to be that a gentle adjustment given whilst you are focused, breathing deeply and relaxed can be very effective…and it's so much nicer to give and receive.

Practice and feedback

In addition to following these guidelines, it's really important to practise giving adjustments and get good feedback, and to be adjusted yourself so you can feel what works and what doesn't. Ideally, go to a workshop to learn adjustments under the guidance of an experienced senior teacher. If that's not possible, choose an experienced yoga practitioner who will give good, honest feedback, and practise until you feel confident and comfortable.

When you start with your 'real' students, start simple and small: choose one small adjustment and just do that. Once you're confident with that, add on one at a time. Enjoy it!

How to choose whom to adjust

When faced with a room full of yoga students all doing different versions of a pose, how do you decide whom to adjust? Are there any guiding principles?

- The first priority is to make sure everyone is safe, so if someone is doing something that looks as if it might lead to injury, that is your priority. Always put safety first.

- Next, if you have someone who is pregnant, prioritise making them safe, supported and looked after (see the earlier section on pregnancy).
- If you know a particular student is working on something, or finds something particularly difficult, always try to be there when they need you.
- Try to ensure that you share your attention with everyone in the class.
- After a while, giving adjustments becomes like another yoga practice: you flow with it, you look up from one adjustment and your body knows who to go to next. Learn to trust your intuition and not the thinking mind.

Making adjustments right for different body types

When you are giving adjustments, it's good to remember that just as there isn't one way of doing a pose that works for all body types, the same is true for adjustments. If you're doing an adjustment and you notice that it's causing the student to overarch their lower back, hunch up their shoulders or do something else that looks unhelpful, try to work out why that's happening and how you can make the adjustment work for their body. If a student is much taller or shorter than you, it's likely that you will have to adapt the 'regular' adjustment. If someone is much taller, try getting in closer and using your body weight more. If someone is much smaller, you may have to go down onto your knees to adjust standing poses. Experiment with them and see what you can work out.

Conclusion

I would love to think that this chapter could empower yoga teachers to start to use and enjoy this beautiful aspect of teaching yoga. My advice would be: if it's something you feel drawn towards, then start to practise. Start with one small, gentle correction and build up slowly from there. Feedback is invaluable, so encourage your students to let you know how it feels. If you can, get yourself to workshops and practise on your friends. Enjoy!

— 9 —

Yoga and Qigong

Mimi Kuo-Deemer

I remember my first experience of *wuji* (Emptiness Stance 无极), qigong's equivalent of Mountain Pose (*Tāḍāsana*). It was 2003, when I was in my early 30s and mainly practising and teaching Vinyasa yoga. The teacher who instructed me into *wuji* was Matthew Cohen, a yogi, martial artist and dancer based in Los Angeles. I liked his approach to movement, so I put aside my uncertainty about qigong and gave it a try. As he talked me into the pose, I placed my feet shoulders' distance apart instead of together. I bent my knees a few inches and dropped my centre of gravity. Rather than lifting my chest and broadening my shoulders, I settled my body and relaxed all the joint spaces. Matthew described *wuji* as the 'shorter, rounder cousin of *Tāḍāsana*', which made me smile. The result of my East Asian *Tāḍāsana* was surprising: my hands felt like sweaty heat lamps and I imagined myself completely rooted into the earth, like a giant redwood tree. Though my legs were shaking by the end (the strength it takes to stand in *wuji* is more than one might imagine), I also felt full of vitality and bright calm.

That first encounter with qigong changed everything for me; I had discovered what it was like to cultivate energy in my body. I also understood that while yoga *āsana* physically extended and stretched my body, energetically, with qigong, I could explore more. In this chapter I'll share some of the ways that yoga and qigong have cross-pollinated in my practice and my teaching of Vinyasa yoga and highlight aspects that I believe can complement and support the ways yoga can be experienced and shared.

What is qigong?

Qigong (气功, pronounced CHEE-GUNG) is a form of energy cultivation. '*Qi*' in Chinese means 'life energy' and '*gong*' 'to cultivate'. It is considered one of the pillars of Chinese medicine but also the basis of all Chinese martial arts, which draws its principles from Daoism and Chan Buddhism.[1] In Daoism and Buddhism, qigong remains the primary means of moving and exercising the body, regulating the breath and calming the mind/heart (*xin* 心) on the path to spiritual awakening. It is therefore a practice that can, at once, be medicinal, martial and spiritual. Though qigong practitioners may emphasise one of these three aspects of qigong, I believe they are inseparable.

Qigong employs a blend of active and dynamic movements, breathing, visualisation and meditation techniques aimed at cultivating healthy *qi* flow through the body's organs and meridians. In Chinese medicine, the organs are described as having distinct physiological functions, such as the heart for circulation and the lungs for respiration. The organs are connected to pathways known as meridians that distribute *qi* through the body. It is believed that the organs and meridians are invested with emotional qualities and spiritual characteristics that can affect a person's health beyond physiological states (see the table later in the chapter).

Qigong adheres to the principle of '*xing ming shuang xiu*', or 'The body's energy, form and spirit are equally refined.' This principle assumes that the body's *qi* can be altered and affected: it has the potential to be clear, healthy and in balance. Because of lifestyle, trauma, injury or stress, however, *qi* can also become stagnant, blocked, diseased, erratic, sluggish, excessive or deficient. In acupuncture, needles are used to clear blockages in the flow of *qi* and support overall health through moving balanced *qi* into the organs and meridians. Much in the same way, qigong works to cultivate healthy *qi* flow where there has been disruption or imbalance, but by using movement, intention, visualisation and breathing techniques.

Like yoga, there are many branches and lineages of qigong. In fact, estimates suggest there are over 7000 forms practised throughout the world today.[2] While that statistic may feel overwhelming, in some ways knowing this can also be a relief. While schools of qigong such as Taiji Chuan (Tai Chi) can be prescriptive in how forms should be executed, for me, knowing there are thousands of forms means that whenever I start thinking I'm doing something 'wrong' I consider whether I have perhaps just created a brilliant new 7001st qigong form!

Qigong's Daoist roots[3]

The belief that the body's *qi* can come into balance is based on observations made by ancient shamanic and Daoist sages. These sages were hired by China's early emperors to observe and report on the patterns of nature. What they discerned was that nature and the universe operate within an order and balance known as *yin* (阴) and *yang* (阳). In its original meaning, *yin* and *yang* was defined as the changing light on a mound as the sun moves across the sky – the transition of shade to sun and back again.[4] In this model, there is no hierarchy. *Yin* and *yang* simply form a complementary opposition and reflect a ceaseless movement of transformation. as maximum *yin* is approached, it changes to *yang*, and vice versa. Governed by something called the Dao,[5] the relationship of *yin* and *yang* give rise to and explain the ongoing rhythms of nature and harmony within the universe.

Since human beings are part of the natural world, the sages concluded that we have the capacity to harmonise with nature rather than to resist it. As a microcosm of the macrocosm, human beings could become one with nature and eventually merge with what the ancient Daoists termed *taiyi* (太一) – a primordial state of great unity or a state of non-differentiated Oneness of the universe.[6] To do this, Daoists were instructed to practise meditation and breathing techniques, as well as to move the body using forms. These forms were known as the *daoyin*, or 'leading and guiding the *qi*' (导引), sometimes called Daoist yoga, and are considered the oldest known styles of qigong. *Daoyin* practices can be traced to scrolls dating back to 168 BC that depicted people stretching, breathing, hopping and imitating animal movements, such as the monkey, dragon, crane and bear. They were described as benefiting health from a wide range of conditions, from flatulence and rheumatism to disturbances to the nervous system and anxiety.[7]

The *daoyin* forms emphasised Daoist principles, such as simplicity, balance, effortlessness and living in harmony with the Dao, often described and translated as 'The Way' or 'The Source'. For myself, these fluid practices are appealing: they help me attune to physical, mental and emotional changes occurring within my body throughout a day or a month, or with the seasonal shifts and turns. Many variants of these early forms are still practised today. Known as the Five Animal Frolics and the Eight Brocades, they are among my favourite practices and remain some of the most popular forms of qigong practice throughout the world.

Yoga and qigong

The connection to the natural world is one of the more compelling narratives for me within both yoga and qigong. In Daoist cosmology and Chinese medicine, there are direct correlations between the seasons, elements, organs and meridian systems and directions. The organs and their related meridians also have associated colours, sounds, odours and emotions (see the table below). Many of the qigong practices today are based on balancing these elements within our bodies, which can in turn balance our physical and emotional states.

Correlative system for the Chinese Five Elements/Phases

Season and element	Direction	Organ and Meridian System	Colour	Emotion
Autumn, Metal	West	Lungs and Large Intestine	White	Dignity, courage/grief and anxiety
Winter, Water	North	Kidneys and Urinary Bladder	Blue/ black	Inner strength, tenacity, confidence/fear and loneliness
Spring, Wood	East	Liver and Gall Bladder	Green	Kindness/anger and jealousy
Summer, Fire	South	Heart, Small Intestine, Triple Heater and Pericardium	Red	Contentment and tranquillity/nervousness and excitability
Late summer, Earth	Centre	Spleen and Stomach	Yellow	Trust, openness, sincerity/ obsessiveness and self-doubt

Yoga practitioners throughout the centuries have also looked to the idea of the natural elements in the world, viewing them as the source of existence, as well as the focus for meditative practice and the path leading to liberation. Yoga traditions from *Sāṃkhya* onwards have given emphasis to the importance of the elements (*tattvas*) of Earth, Water, Fire, Wind and Ether as the foundations for practices leading to liberation.

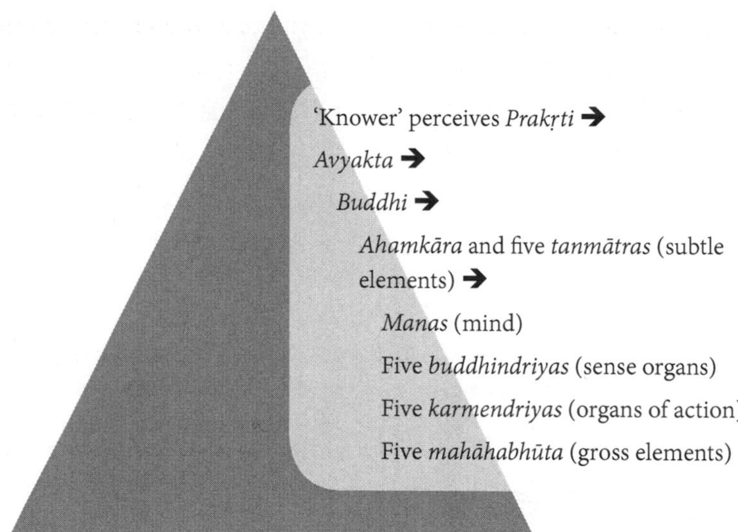

***SAṂKHYAN* MODEL OF THE MATERIAL WORLD**

While both disciplines give emphasis to elemental qualities and characteristics within the natural world, how they engage with these elements remains distinct.

Water, Earth and Fire

In Daoism, water is believed to be present at the beginning and end of all things. Because of this, it is often equated to the eternal and universal Dao.[8] The early Daoists also believed that the body – including blood, bones, essence, thoughts and spirit – are all part of the fluid, watery matrix that is the Dao.[9] The Daoist text of the *Tao Te Ching*, describes water:[10]

> *Nothing in the world*
> *is as soft and yielding as water*
> *Yet for overcoming the hard and inflexible,*
> *nothing can surpass it.*
> *The soft overcomes the hard;*
> *the gentle overcomes the rigid.*
> *Everyone knows this is true,*
> *but few can put it into practice.*[11]

From a Daoist viewpoint, harmonising the fluids and energies of our own mind and body allows us to become one with the flowing energies of nature and the universe. Over time and through experimentation, Daoists found the most effective way to do this was through the soft, gentle movements and smooth, deep breathing often associated with qigong today.

From a physiological perspective, qigong's smooth, flowing movements and breathing patterns are highly therapeutic to the body's bones and joints. When movements are jerky and uncontrolled, breathing is jerky and uncontrolled. A jagged, shallow breath can create muscular tension, which in turn can obstruct the circulation of *qi* through the body. Additionally, these factors when compounded, can lead to strain in tendons, ligaments and joints. When movements are rhythmic and steady, we can avoid such imbalances and we facilitate the healthy flow of synovial fluid, which protects and cushions most of the body's joints.[12] Synovial fluid reduces friction between bones and can help reduce arthritis and inflammation. It also provides nutrients and oxygen to a joint's cartilage layer, which receives no blood flow of its own and therefore relies on a fresh supply of synovial fluid to stay healthy. Fluid movements also support the healthy circulation of blood and *qi*, which in turn help balance the body's energy and maintain its natural healing potential.[13]

There is also an emphasis in the early Daoist beliefs on the '*yin*' characteristic of being more grounded and feminine and harnessing receptivity as a source of strength. Again, in the *Tao Te Ching*, it is written that:

> *The heavy is the root of the light;*
> *The still is the lord of the restless...*
> *If light, then the root is lost;*
> *If restless, then the lord is lost...*
> *Know the male*
> *But keep to the role of the female...*
> *Know the white*
> *But keep to the role of the black.*[14]

The emphasis on water and the grounded qualities of yin from Daoism translate what one American qigong teacher, Kenneth Cohen, describes as *Strong as the Mountain, Supple as Water.*[15] Patterned on the stability of the earth and the unbroken and continuous qualities of wind and water, qigong tends to employ steady, soft, circular movements and shapes.

In yogic practices, a different story unfolds. Fire and worship of Agni[16] is described in the *Upaniṣads* as the means for 'the attainment of an endless world'.[17] Though earth and water figure importantly in the yoga tradition, fire-based practices stand out as the most significant.[18] Moreover, a yogi's transformation is primarily achieved through *tapas,* or a disciplined, heated effort that produces more heat.[19] Through *tapas,* yogis believed that *karma* (one's action) becomes purified until the impure aspects of the individual Self can unite with the pure and eternal Self that is Brahman. The emphasis on *tapas* has been translated into a number of popular forms of yoga today such as Ashtanga, Vinyasa, Bikram and hot yoga that increase heat by means of vigorous effort.

Personally, I find the Daoist and yogic narratives equally compelling. Pretty much every day, I will do a variation of a sun salutation as part of my yoga practice and build into more dynamic sequences involving backbends, twists, forward folds and inversions. I love the heat, extension and vitality I feel from a dynamic yoga practice. Yet I also value cultivating smooth, fluid and steady movement patterns within the intensity of *āsana.* Leaving the divergent soteriological goals of qigong and yoga aside, from my experience, integrating aspects of qigong into my yoga practice has granted me far more balance, fluidity and cohesion in how I approach *āsana.*

Applying qigong concepts to yoga

Generally speaking, in yoga *āsana* movements of the body tend to exhibit in more linear, straight lines, while the emphasis in qigong is on rounder, more spherical shapes. For example, if you consider Triangle Pose (*Trikoṇāsana*), the spine extends in two directions through the crown of the head and tailbone, and the limbs reach out in straight lines from the ground upward as well as from the centre of the body outward. *Tāḍāsana* can also emphasise a more linear orientation of the body: the kneecaps lift to strengthen and lengthen the legs, and the shoulders draw back and the chest forward to support the lengthening of the spine. While Triangle Pose can certainly be stable, the overall shape – when contrasted to something like qigong's Dragon – is more linear.

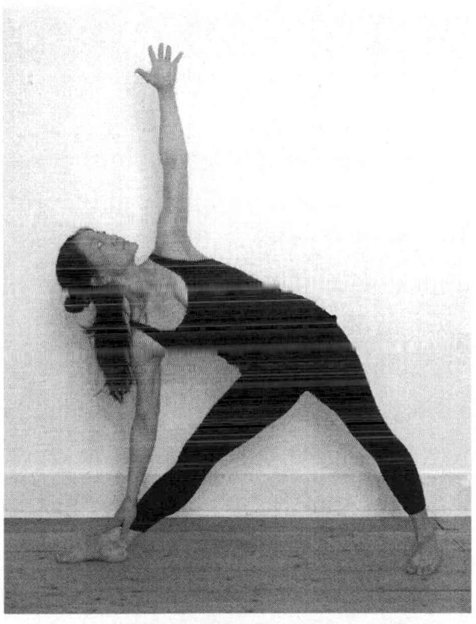

TRIANGLE POSE

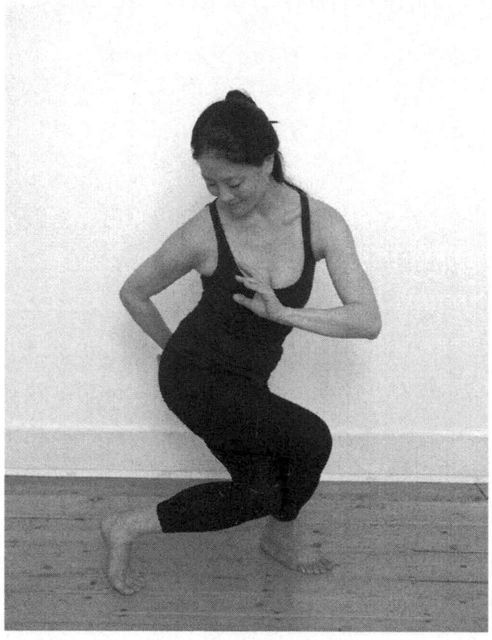

DRAGON

When the circular qualities of qigong are introduced into the more linear shapes in yoga *āsana*, new insights can be made about ways to experience the same pose through a different emphasis and intention. In this following section, I will explore how yoga and qigong work with similar concepts but conceive of them in distinct ways. I'll also illustrate how certain ideas from qigong such as *chen* (rooting, sinking), *yi* (intention) and *wuwei* (effortless effort) can support the ways we potentially practise, teach and share yoga.

Chen: sinking into the earth

The first concept, *chen* (to go deep, root, submerge 沉), means to give weight into the earth. The character for *chen* contains the radicals for water, as well as a roof and a table. Considering water's associated qualities of strength and eternal Oneness that is the Dao, when one initiates *chen*, one is invited to immerse oneself deeply and sink beneath the surface of everyday experience so as to gain wisdom and greater insight.

In qigong, *chen* involves an active giving of weight into the earth. It is similar to the image of trees establishing stability through root systems reaching down into the earth that then support the upward growth and expansion of branches and leaves towards the sky. The execution of *chen*, however, is also different from the action of rooting in the action of the feet in *Pada Bandha* (foot seal) from yoga. Instead of rooting through the feet and ankles, with *chen* the knees will also bend, root and 'sink' downward. In addition, when one takes *chen*, the sacrum will extend the spine downwards, rather than the tailbone, for example, as one might instruct in yoga. This creates a lower centre of gravity that lends an increased stability and rootedness. Though there is always an upward reach through the spine from the crown, overall there is a lower centre of gravity and more active giving of weight into the earth.

This concept of *chen* can be useful in a number of instances for yoga practitioners. One example may be where a student feels rickety and unsteady, such as in balance poses like Half Moon Pose (*Ardha Candrāsana*). By keeping the standing leg knee more bent and the centre of weight lower to the earth, a student may feel more stable. Another helpful application may be when initiating *chen* in the body before moving forwards or backwards to provide momentum that supports a rebound and reach into space. This is similar to what basketball players, dancers and free runners use as a resource to jump off the ground and into the air. The feeling of rooting may also find expression through the dynamic and fluid transitions of Low Plank (*Caturaṅga*) into Upward Facing Dog (*Urdhva Mukha Svanāsana*) of a *vinyāsa*, where the body's momentum can oscillate between *chen* (yielding), rebounding and reaching.

As a teacher, *chen* can also be valuable when establishing greater steadiness in your body before assisting your students in a pose. Try this with a co-teacher or friend to test each other's stability: when standing in a conventional *Tāḍāsana* have your partner gently push you off-centre. Then try standing with the feeling of *chen* through your body. When your partner gently pushes you again, you may observe how much steadier you are and how much harder it is to knock you off balance. The active giving of weight into the earth can be a resourceful and grounding experience that benefits you and your student.

Yi (intention) directs *qi*

In qigong, the concept of *yi* (intention, 意) is the primary way in which energy (*qi*) can be experienced and affected. *Yi* is believed to move, direct and refine *qi* through the body. In Chinese there is a saying: 'When the *yi* arrives, the *qi* arrives' (*yi dao, qi dao*). This is a difficult concept for some to wrap their heads around intellectually because energy is something felt rather than logically reasoned. Thus, simply reading about how intention can affect our energy will never replace experiencing and feeling how it unfolds. With this in mind, try this exercise.

HOW *YI* (INTENTION) CAN DIRECT *QI*

- Take your hands out to the side, turn your palms upward and lift them overhead. Notice the action of lifting. Release them back down, and also notice what the quality of movement is like.
- Now take your hands out to the side, turn your palms upward and imagine that a butterfly lands in the palm of each hand. With the butterflies there, lift your hands overhead with the intention of keeping your rare and precious passengers still on your hands. Notice what the quality of movement is. Then release your hands back down, still with the butterflies on your palms, remaining aware of how your body moves.

- Finally, take your hands out to the side, turn your palms upward, and imagine that your hands are holding heavy, ripe papayas that are rather difficult to lift up. Notice resistance you feel as the hands and arms lift overhead. When you release the hands, turn your palms out and down, imagining there's a huge beach ball beneath them that you're trying to push underwater. Notice how the arms and hands move and whether you can feel resistance.

Chances are, if you did this exercise, you'll have figured out that with a butterfly in the palm of the hand, the movement slowed down and became steadier, more graceful and possibly more receptive. You may have also noticed with the image of something heavy like a papaya in each hand that the movement quality also changed. This is one way how our *yi* (intention) can affect how we experience *qi* (energy): in using the intention to ensure the butterfly is not disturbed or the intention that the ball is submerged beneath the water, we can create a specific quality to any movement.

In Chinese, the character for *yi* (intention, 意) is formed using the radicals for the heart, the sun and the verb to establish or stand. When we integrate the concept of *yi* into any action, we can think of it as calling on our heart and the light of the sun to help us cultivate clear positions and directions. This is similar to *saṅkalpa* in yoga, which means intention but can also be understood as being formed from the root words *san*, meaning 'formed in the heart', and *kalpa*, meaning 'a way to proceed'. *Saṅkalpa* is frequently introduced into yoga classes, but not necessarily through the use of intentions and visualisations for how to specifically move or direct *prāṇa* or *qi*.

In a number of specific qigong forms, the names of the forms are themselves invitations to use visualisations and intention, such as 'Moving Clouds', 'Pushing Waves' or 'Drawing the Bow'. When I teach yoga, I often integrate the use of *yi* by incorporating visualisations to affect and direct the intention within an *āsana* or sequence.

Visualisations can give any action depth and richness beyond the movement itself. I often like to use imagery to support ease in movement, particularly through transitions. Normally, if I instruct a class to bring the foot forward from a Downdog Split into a runner's lunge, the transition can sound clunky and loud. If I add the intention to 'moon land' the lunging foot forward to the floor, or step it forward as though it were a feather landing on the earth, the movements become far more integrated. In fact, I rarely hear a peep in the transition.

Another way I integrate *yi* in classes is to instruct them to do what is called a 'clearing, filling and sealing' practice. Near the beginning of class or as part of a sun salutation series, I might have students standing in *Tāḍāsana* or *wuji* and then raise their arms overhead, gathering qualities of tightness, tension or constriction in the body. I'll then have them bend the elbows, turning the palms towards the earth and lower the hands down slowly to clear out tension in their eyes and jaw; as they pass lower down I may mention how they can clear out tightness in their shoulders, chest or back. I'll follow with filling something like sunlight or clarity and finish with sealing it all in to the body. An illustrated example of a 'clearing, filling and sealing' practice is given later in the chapter.

Yi (intention), *prāṇa* and *qi*

The role of *yi* is also helpful in understanding how *prāṇa* and *qi*, both considered vital energy within yoga and qigong respectively, can be understood as similar yet distinct concepts. In yoga, *prāṇa* is understood to move through the pathways of the body, known as the *naḍis*. The most important *naḍis* are the *ida* (left feminine, lunar channel), *pingala* (right masculine, solar channel) and *suṣumnā* (central channel). *Chakras* are also understood to manifest where these three *naḍis* intersect in whirling vortices of energy. *Prāṇa* also manifests in different forms known as the *vāyus*, or winds, that comprise the energy of a pranic body.[20] All these *vāyus* serve different functions in the body and all can become deficient or excessive. The healthy function of *prāṇa* in the body can be positively or negatively affected by what we eat, think, do or absorb from our environment.

Qi also moves into the body via the breath and follows pathways known as meridians that connect to organs. There are also different types of *qi* that manifest in the body as breath, food, original, internal, external, nutritive and protective *qi*.[21] There are also three main channels that are similar to the location and associated qualities of yoga's *ida*, *pingala*, and *suṣumnā* known as the *renmai* (*yin*, feminine, receptive governing meridian), *dumai* (*yang*, masculine, active governing meridian) and *chongmai* (central, penetrating meridian). In qigong, three reservoirs of energy are also located along the central body called the lower, middle and upper *dantian*. While there are certainly many potential areas of overlap in how *qi* and *prāṇa* can be understood in yoga and qigong, the two approach the function and practices of energy flow in the body distinctly, particularly with regard to *yi* (intention).

Though *prāṇa* may in fact be directed by intention, it is not necessarily at the forefront of practices such as *prāṇāyāma*. Instead, *prāṇāyāma* is often done in an effort to control the breath, often (but not always)[22] through force.[23] Throughout most of yogic history, it has been associated with *tapas*, or the heated forms of ascetic practice.[24] Perhaps because of its association with strong, heating practices, *prāṇāyāma* has often been considered dangerous. Indeed, when the Buddha tried breath control, he described it as bringing about a 'painful feeling' that was like 'stabbing a cow's stomach with a sharp butcher's knife' or like 'extreme winds' slashing his head 'as if a strong man were attacking my head with a sharp sword' before finally giving up the practice' (*Majjhimanikāya* I:9).[25]

Breathing practices are also used in qigong but, in order to affect the *qi*, one uses visualisations and intention (*yi)* in breathing rather than heat or force. In fact, visualisations of *qi* flow are some of my go-to qigong practices when I'm feeling sick or cannot do my regular *āsana* practice. One of my favourites is a gemstone visualisation, which uses the colours associated with organs and relates them to precious stones.

I often do this visualisation (below) when I feel I'm on the brink of getting a cold or cough, and nine out of ten times I'll avoid getting sick.

Gemstone qigong visualisation practice

The practice involves breathing a colour of a precious gemstone into each organ and exhaling what dulls the shine of that colour. The practice is inspired by Kenneth Cohen, but it is a well-known Daoist healing technique.

For the lungs, the colour to breathe in is a pure diamond white. Exhale what dulls the brilliance of the diamond shine. For the kidneys, the colour is sapphire blue; again, exhale what limits the colour from shining its deep, splendid blue. For the liver, the colour is emerald green; the heart, ruby red; and the spleen, topaz orange. With each organ, exhale what dulls the richness of the colour shining through. Once you have brought breath and a richer colour of precious gemstones to each organ, imagine all the gemstones of your organs shining beautifully inside your body, vibrant and alive.

Wuwei: effortless effort

Wuwei (无为), or effortless effort, is a concept central to Daoist beliefs. It translates directly as 'without action' or 'without effort'. It can also suggest that one uses an economy of effort: only as much as is necessary and no more than you need. With *wuwei*, there is also a quality of naturalism implied. When nothing is forced, a natural harmony can be felt that enables us to resist and tense less against the free flow of experience. This does not mean that nothing happens and we don't do anything, but by interfering and meddling less, we learn to see beyond the necessity of constantly trying to 'do' and 'be' something. This allows us to relax into the possibility of allowing and receiving more freely. As the *Tao Te Ching* describes:

We join the spokes together in a wheel,
But it is the centre hole
That makes the wagon move.
We shape clay into a pot,
But it is the emptiness inside
That holds whatever we want.
We hammer wood for a house,
But it is the inner space
That makes it liveable.
We work with being,
But non-being is what we use.[26]

When I introduce concepts such as *wuwei* into yoga classes, it is often in the context of when students begin to struggle or tense in postures. A gentle reminder of only using what's necessary and softening unnecessary force or gripping can often transform how students experience their practice.

Weaving qigong forms and sequences into a yoga class

Over the years, many of my students have told me that they enjoy the qigong concepts and forms that I'll weave into my Vinyasa Flow classes. What are the ways I introduce elements of qigong? During a standing pose sequence, I might have students explore a less rigid version of *Trikoṇāsana* or *Vīrabhadrāsana II* by alternating bending the front and *back* knee to feel more grounded and steady (*chen*) through the legs into the pelvis. In poses such as Warrior Two, I will invite students to do variations of 'crane flying' (see the following section). Thus, without scaring my students away by completely breaking from the familiarity of yoga forms and functions, I open up some ground for sensing into new ways to meet a pose through different movement qualities derived from qigong.

While there are infinitely creative ways to introduce aspects of qigong practices and forms into yoga, I will offer two primary concepts that may be safe and accessible for yourself and your students.

Fire/yang-based practices, forms and sequences

The postures below are forms that can often be threaded into Vinyasa Flow sequences or stand alone within the context of a class.

CRANE FLYING

Starting in *Vīrabhadrāsana II*, inhale and retract the elbows and hands in; exhale, extend the hands with the palms turned out away from you. Repeat two to three times.

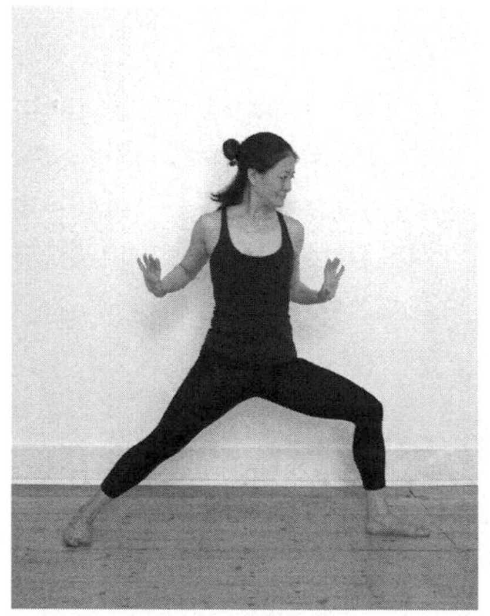

CRANE FLYING 1

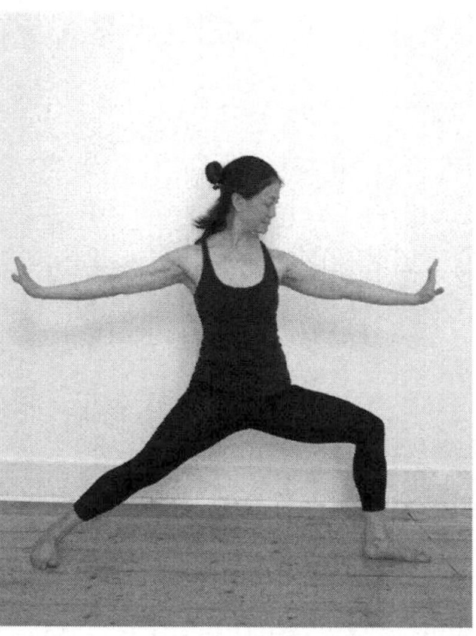

CRANE FLYING 2

CRANE

Feet stand heels together, toes out. Fingertips touch the thumbs and curl in towards your wrists as you inhale and lift the hands to the level of the shoulders, bending the knees. Exhale, release the hands out and down. Repeat three to six times.

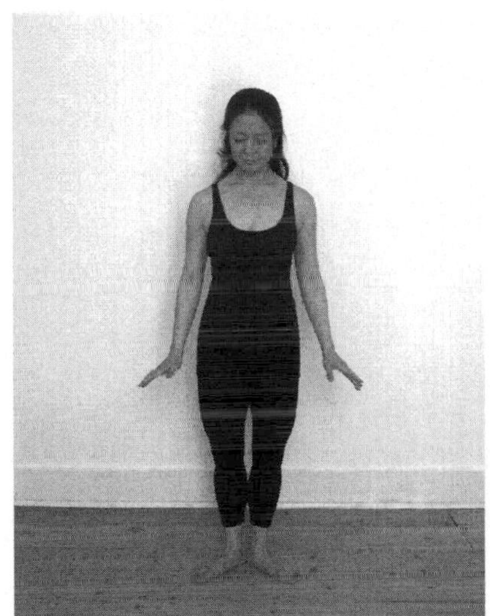

CRANE 1

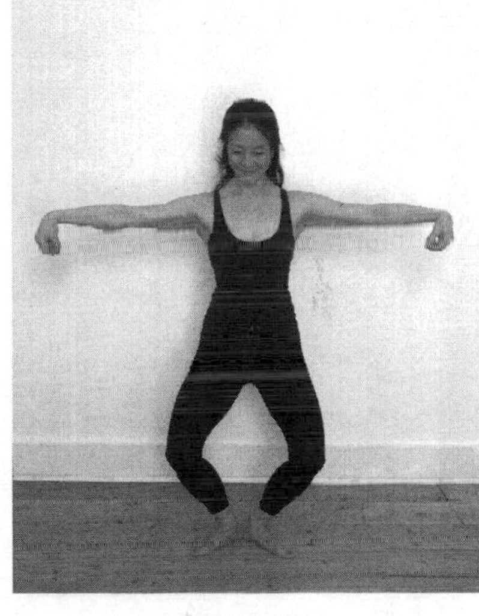

CRANE 2

This can be used to prepare the wrists for weight-bearing and arm balancing as part of the sun salutations (e.g. from *Tādāsana*).

HORSE STANCE

Stand the feet three to four feet apart, toes turned out slightly and knees bent. The arms can be either extended to the side (see the image on the left) or rounded forward with the elbows soft and shoulders relaxed (see the image on the right).

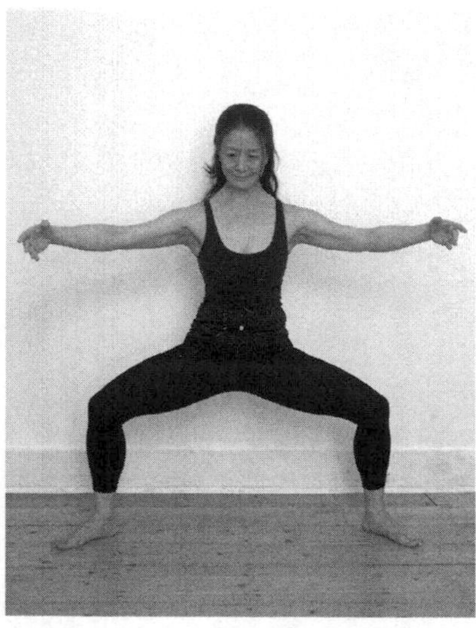

HORSE STANCE 1

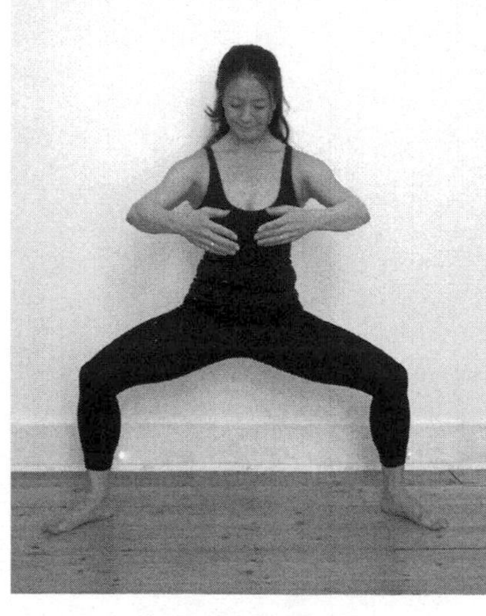

HORSE STANCE 2

Horse Stance can be used before or after Warrior Two (*Vīrabhadrāsana II)* or Exalted/Reverse Warrior or Standing Wide Leg Forward Fold Pose (*Prasārita Padottanāsana*).

TAMING THE TIGER

The legs are both bent with the feet turned out. The back leg carries 60–70 per cent of the body's weight, and the front leg 30–40 per cent. The hands are low and facing the front leg as though about to tame a tiger pouncing.

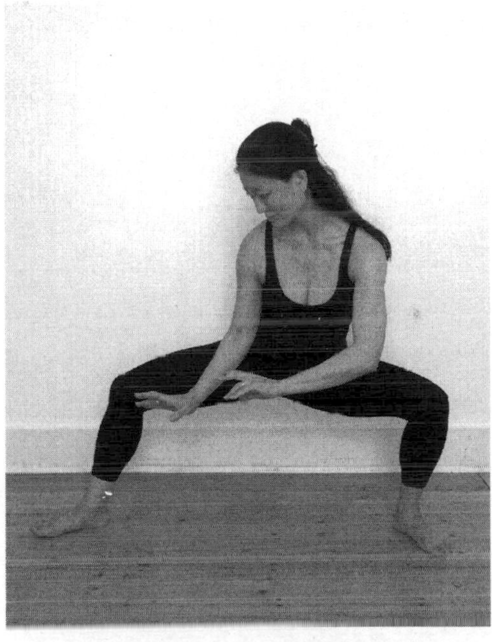

TAMING THE TIGER

This can be introduced before or after Warrior Two (*Vīrabhadrāsana II*) or Exalted/Reverse Warrior.

DRAGON

Standing on the right foot, the left foot steps diagonally behind the front leg with the heel lifted. The right hand fingers all touch the thumb and the back of the hand is placed on the sacrum as though it is a dragon's tail. The left hand is soft in front of the chest, elbow bent. With the knees bending, the body rotates towards the right while keeping the crown lifted and the tailbone reaching back and down. Repeat on the left.

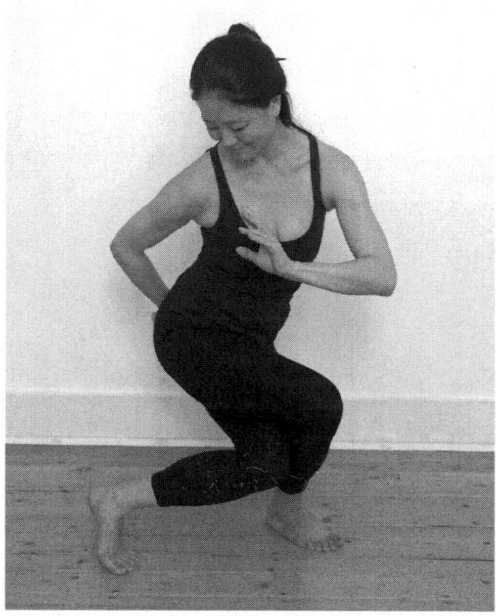

DRAGON

This can be included with standing poses. One particular transition I love is from Eagle Pose (*Garudāsana*) into Dragon.

THROWING THE FISHING NET

From Horse Stance, the arms reach overhead and the hands hold an imaginary fishing net that you throw 360 degrees around. Circle one direction three to five times and then repeat by circling the other direction.

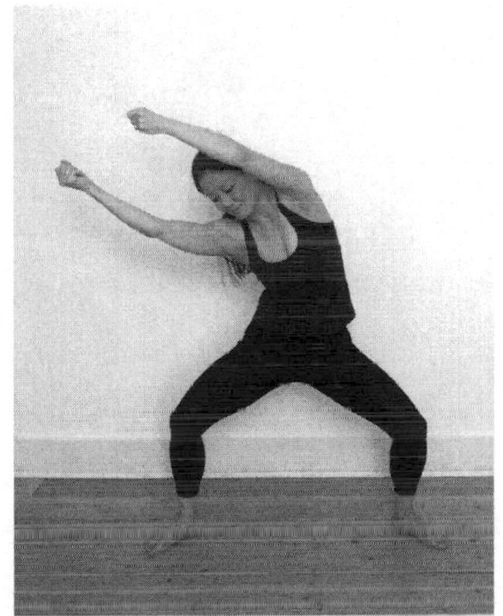

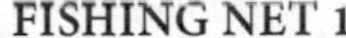

FISHING NET 1

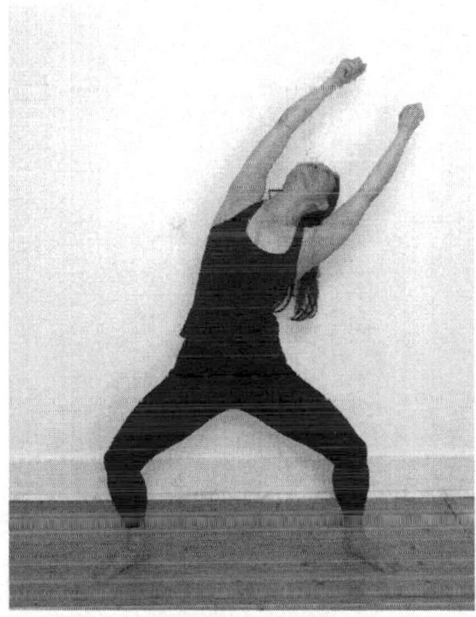

FISHING NET 2

This can be used from Horse Stance or introduced before or after Standing Wide Leg Forward Fold Pose (*Prasārita Padottanāsana*).

BIRD NESTING

From Horse Stance, bend the right knee; use the right hand to make a 'bird' and the left to make a 'nest'. Weight shift and bend the left knee, straightening the right leg. Shift the nest down and around to the other side, making a bird with that hand and a nest with the other hand. Weight shift the body and change legs, repeat on the second side. This can be repeated three to five times.

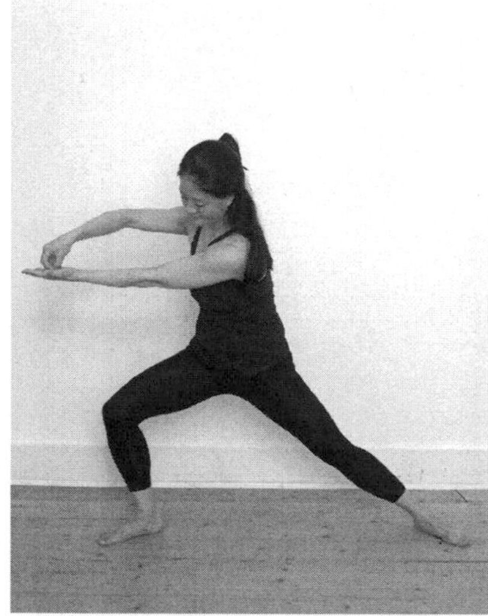

BIRD NESTING 1

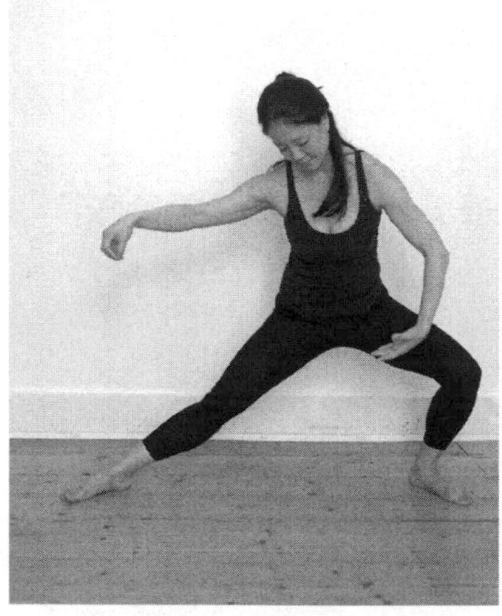

BIRD NESTING 2

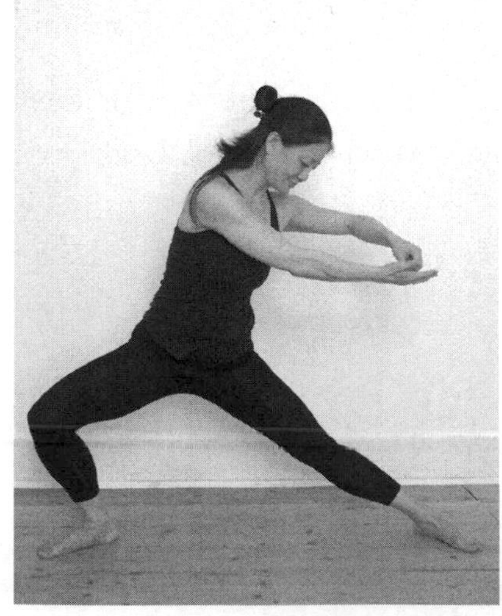

BIRD NESTING 3

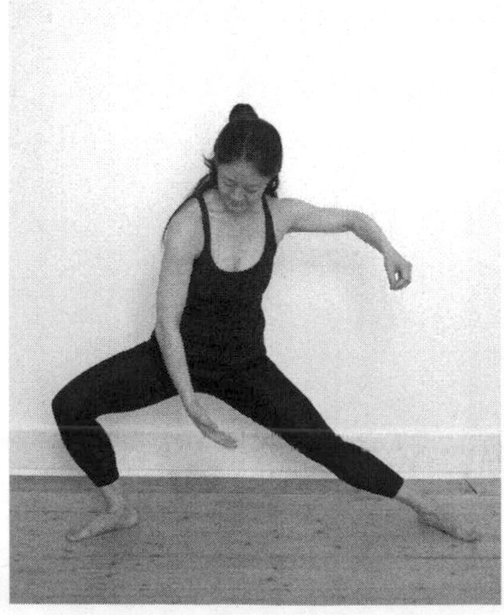

BIRD NESTING 4

This sequence can be used before or after Horse Stance, Warrior Two (*Vīrabhadrāsana II*), Exalted/Reverse Warrior, or Standing Spread Leg Forward Fold Pose (*Prasārita Padottanāsana*).

Water/yin-based practices and forms

CLEARING, FILLING, SEALING

The hands reach out to the sides, palms turned up, inhaling. Once the hands are over the head, the elbows bend, the middle fingers point towards each other and the hands then pass down in front of the body.

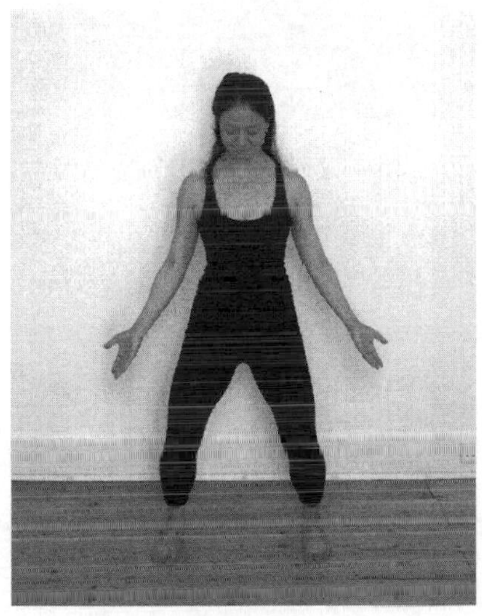

CLEARING 1

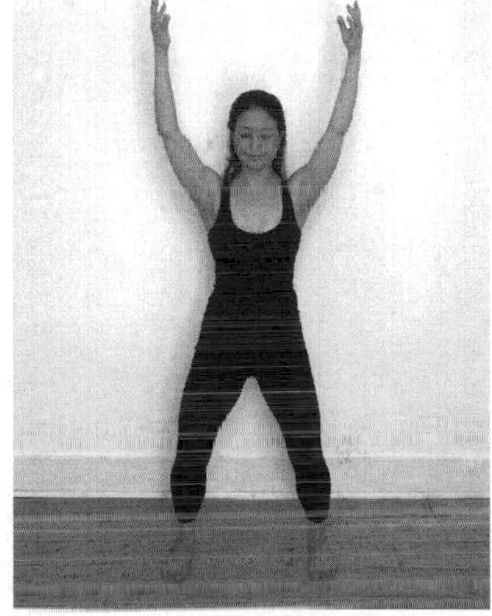

CLEARING 2

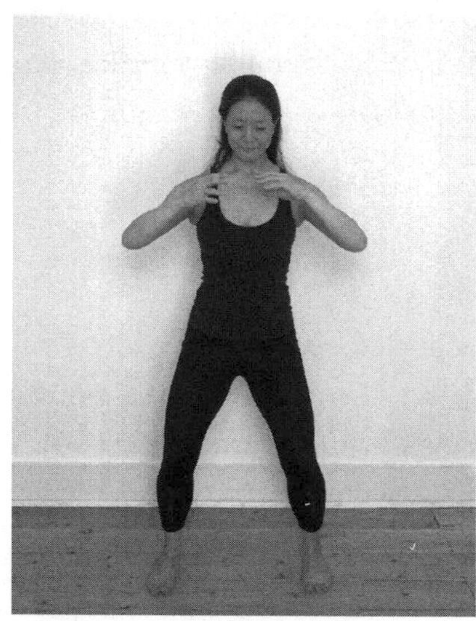

CLEARING 3

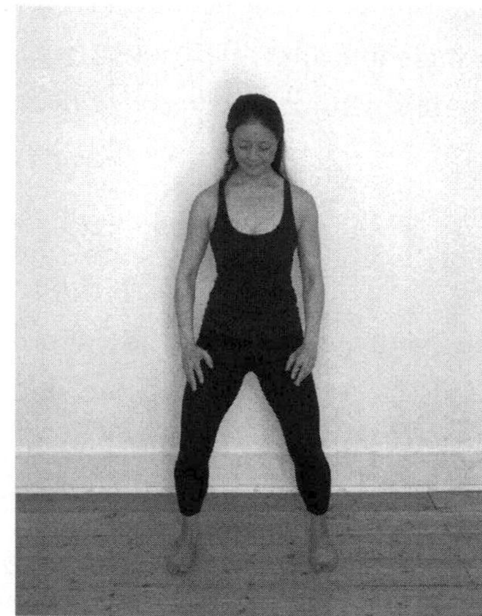

CLEARING 4

This sequence can be introduced near the beginning of class as part of an opening or Sun Salute. This works strongly with *yi* (intention). The movements are repeated between one and three times with different intentions. You can start with clearing away things such as:

- sleepiness, sluggishness, lethargy or dullness
- tension, tightness, contraction or discomfort in the physical body
- negative thoughts, irritation, impatience, anxiety, fear.

Then follow with filling with qualities such as:

- clarity, light, energy, wakefulness
- spaciousness, ease, comfort
- positive thoughts, kindness, patience, compassion, love.

PARTING CLOUDS

Inhale and take the hands in towards the chest, rolling them in and then down, exhaling and moving the palms away from the body to part clouds.

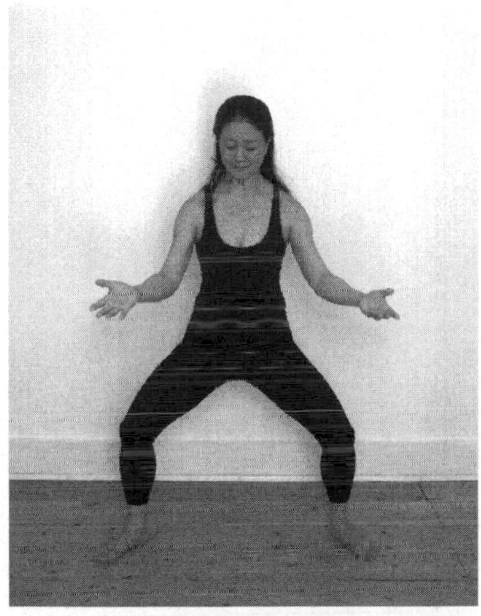

PARTING CLOUDS 1

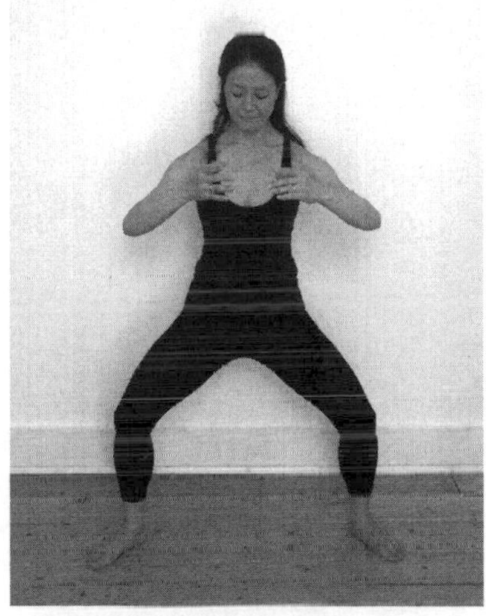

PARTING CLOUDS 2

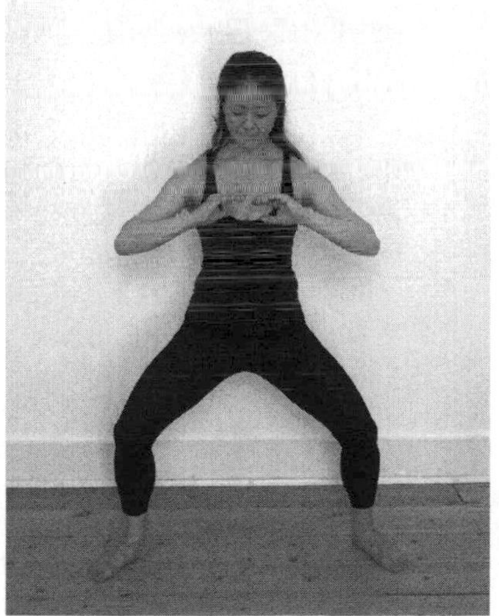

PARTING CLOUDS 3

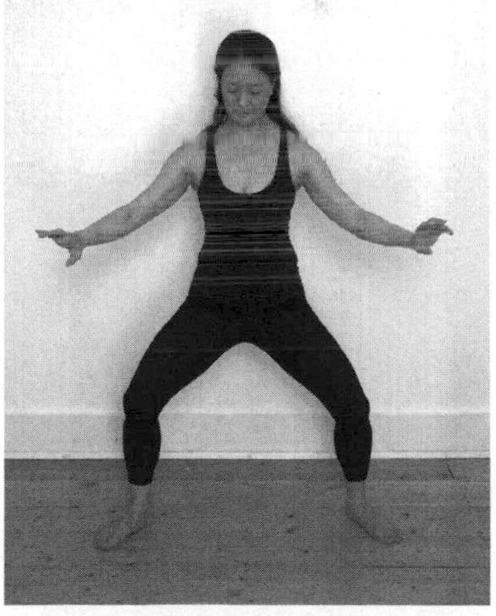

PARTING CLOUDS 4

This can be used any time in standing or from Horse Stance.

ETHERIC CLEANSING

From Horse Stance, take one hand to the opposite arm, keeping the hand a few inches from the skin. Keep the hand a few inches from the skin as you clear up the outer arm to the shoulder, then down the inner arm to the palm. Repeat with the other arm, then move to both hands clearing along one leg and then the other.

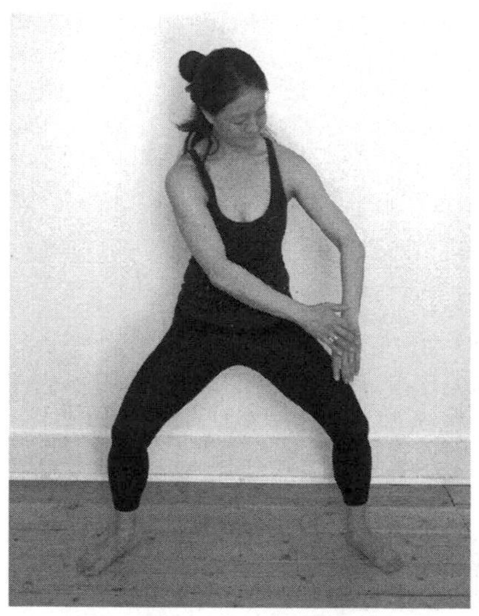

ETHERIC CLEANSING 1

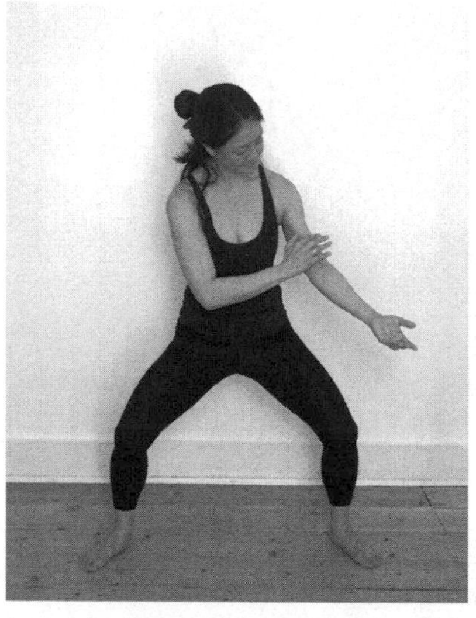

ETHERIC CLEANSING 2

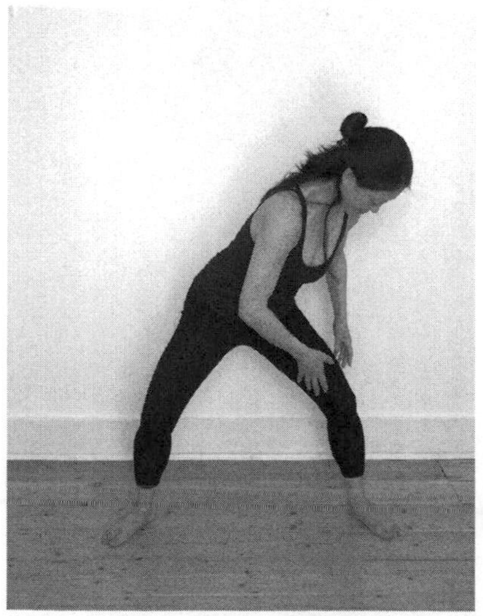

ETHERIC CLEANSING 3

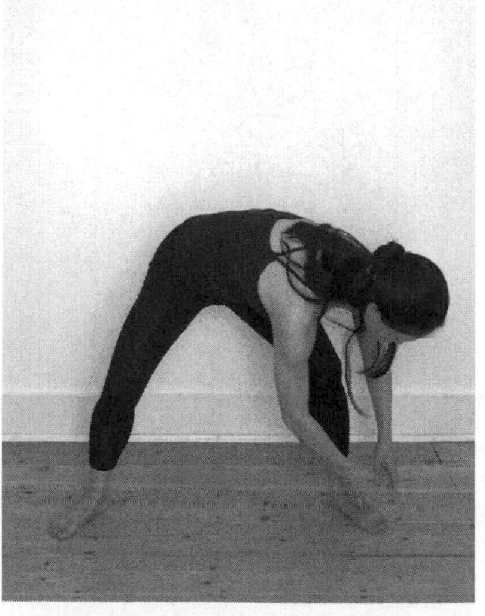

ETHERIC CLEANSING 4

This can be used after standing poses and can provide a good transition to seated postures.

HANDS TO HEART

Breathing normally, take the palms out to the sides and then exhale, lower the chin and bend the elbows in, resting one hand over the other on the centre of the chest.

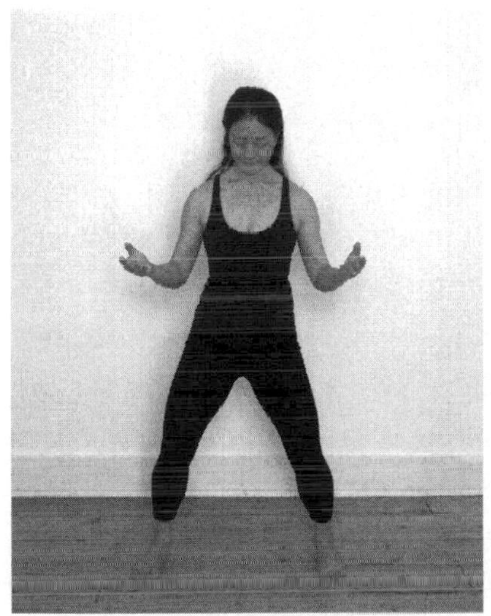

HANDS TO HEART 1

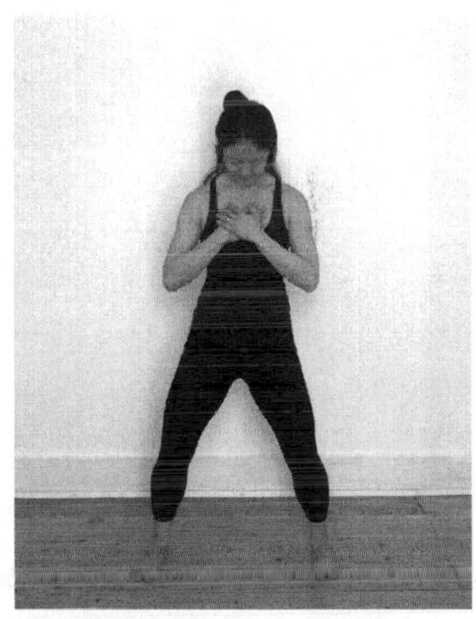

HANDS TO HEART 2

This is a very good practice to be used before or after backbends.

Concluding comments: freedom from form

Within the limitations of this short chapter on yoga and qigong, I have outlined a few primary concepts that I have found helpful in the ways I bring qigong into my yoga practice and teaching. In exploring this integration, perhaps some readers may raise eyebrows at my willingness to break from form and expand the traditions of yoga into lineage-less territories. My personal view of yoga, however, is that it is a process that helps expand consciousness. It heightens awareness and invites anyone willing to dedicate the time and energy to its practice to begin to live more in the light of our own understanding. This means establishing a degree of freedom from orthodoxy and moving beyond the limitations of what we think we know or assume to be correct. In a sense, it is a process that invites me to explore my willingness to embrace the ambiguous, mysterious and unknown. Paradoxically, by embracing this degree of uncertainty and not-knowing, I feel closer to the heart of both yoga and the Dao.

Additional reading

As introductions to qigong and Chinese medicine's basic theories, some accessible yet highly informative books are Kenneth Cohen's *The Way of Qigong: The Art and Science of Chinese Energy Healing* (1997, Ballantine Books) and Gail Richstein's *Wood Becomes Water: Chinese Medicine in Everyday Life* (1998, Kodansha). For a poetic introduction to Daoism, read Stephen Mitchell's translation of the *Tao Te Ching* (1988, Harper Perenial Modern Classics). For an enjoyable jaunt into Daoism and Chan Buddhism, Bill Porter's *Road to Heaven: Encounters with Chinese Hermits* (1993, Mercury House) is one of my all-time favourite books. For more academic and historical understandings of Daoism, I suggest Kristofer Schipper's *The Taoist Body* (1993, University of California Press).

Online resources

I have a few qigong practices available on YouTube:

- Eight Brocades Qigong Practice:
www.youtube.com/watch?v=3K-0JpiJu-o&t=1s
- Five Elements Qigong Practice:
www.youtube.com/watch?v=_6Y8QSVyYhM
- Bone Marrow Cleanse Qigong Practice:
www.youtube.com/watch?v=HbWfnlolF9M&t=68s.

I also have a number of classes that are qigong, yoga or yoga/qigong integrations available on www.movementformodernlife.com.

Notes

1 Chan Buddhism is a school of Mahayana Buddhism that combines Daoist beliefs. The monk Bodhidharma is credited for bringing Chan to China in the fifth or sixth century CE. During the Tang Dynasty (618–907 CE), Chan Buddhism spread to Japan and became Zen.

2 Cohen, K. (2005) *The Essential Qigong Training Guide: Strong as the Mountain, Supple as Water.* Colorado: Sounds True. p.5.

3 Throughout Chinese history, Daoism also evolved much in tandem with the philosophy of Confucianism. Confucianism's primary contribution to qigong is an emphasis on intellectual and mental training, applied through the arts as well as anything involving mental focus. Qigong has also been influenced by Buddhism, beginning in the second century CE and continuing through the Tang Dynasty. The Shaolin Temple, for example, is a Buddhist monastery where some of China's most popular qigong forms and martial arts were developed.

4 Schipper, K. (1993) *The Taoist Body*. Trans. K. C. Duval. London: University of California Press. p.35.

5 The Dao is described as 'The Way' but also that which cannot be named and is yet eternally present and real (*Tao Te Ching*, chapter 1).

6 Kohn, L. (1989) 'Guarding the One.' In *Taoist Meditation and Longevity Techniques*. Ann Arbor: Center for Chinese Studies, The University of Michigan. p.18.

7 Cohen, K. (1997) *The Way of Qigong. The Art and Science of Chinese Energy Healing*. New York: Ballantine Books. p.18.

8 Wong, E. (2015) *Being Taoist: Wisdom for Living a Balanced Life*. Boston and London: Shambala Publications. pp.19–20.

9 Ishida, H. (1989) 'Body and Mind: The Chinese Perspective.' In L. Kohn (ed.) *Taoist Meditation and Longevity Techniques*. Ann Arbor: Center for Chinese Studies, The University of Michigan. pp.41–71.

10 *Dao De Jing* is the same as *Tao Te Ching*, and Lao Tzu is the same as Lao Zi; the spelling varies depending on whether the Romanisation of characters follows pinyin or Wade–Giles guidelines.

11 Mitchell, S. (1988) *Tao Te Ching: A New English Version, with Forward and Notes by Stephen Mitchell.* New York: Harper Perenial Modern Classics. Chapter 78.

12 The exceptions are the sacroiliac joint and the intervertebral discs (between the vertebrae).

13 Frantzis, B. (2008) *Dragon and Tiger Medical Qigong, Volume I: Health and Energy in Seven Simple Movements*. Berkeley: North Atlantic Books. p.2.

14 Lao Tzu (1963) *Tao Te Ching*, translated by D.C. Lau. London: Penguin Books. Chapter 26 and 27, p.83, p.85.

15 Cohen 2005.

16 Agni is the Vedic god of fire, which is worshipped in Vedic, Brahmanic and yogic rituals as a deity but also the representative of sacred and continuing life.

17 *Kaṭha Upaniṣads* I.14–15.

18 All the Great Elements of Water, Earth, Fire, Wind and Ether were used as meditative and ritual acts leading to liberation, but fire emerged in the Vedic texts as the most central and important (Frauwallner, E. (1984) *History of Indian Philosophy Vol – I.* Delhi: Motilal Banarsidass Publishers Private Limited. pp.27–75).

19 Kaelber, W. O. (1989) *Tapta Mārga: Asceticism and Initiation in Vedic India.* Delhi: Sri Satguru Publications.

20 There are five *vāyus*: *vyāna vāyu* (moves through the whole body); *udāna vāyu* (moves from the throat upward); *prāṇa vāyu* (moves between the diaphragm and throat); *samāna vāyu* (moves from the navel to the diaphragm); and *apāna vāyu* (moves below the navel).

21 Cohen 1997, p.36.

22 James Mallinson and Mark Singleton in *Roots of Yoga* (2017 p.128, London: Penguin) define *prāṇāyāma* as 'breath control', but Richard Rosen in *The Yoga of Breath: A Step-by-Step Guide to Pranayama* (2002, p.19, Boston and London: Shambala Publications) suggests that *prāṇāyāma* can just as easily be understood as the 'process of expanding our usually small reservoir of prana by lengthening, directing, and regulating the movement of the breath and then limiting or restraining the increased pranic energy in the body-mind'.

23 Mallinson and Singleton 2017, pp.127–170.

24 Mallinson and Singleton 2017, p.127.

25 *Majjhimanikāya I*, Book 9. Trans. J. Mallinson and M. Singleton (2017) *The Roots of Yoga.* London: Penguin. p.138.

26 Trans. Mitchell 1988, Chapter 11.

— 10 —

Āyurvedic Approach — *Yoga with an Āyurvedic Approach*

Tarik Dervish

The sea of yoga is so vast and amorphous that it has been able to withstand the test of time and continually reinvent itself to suit the needs of its captors. It speaks in all tongues and moulds itself to the minds of all who truly seek its essence because its true language actually has no cultural, religious or social boundaries. It will become whatever you want it to if it means you will be inspired enough to engage with it. That is because its truth lies in the mystery of life. The mystery that we are all trying to unravel through our bodies, minds and hearts. The mystery always starts with the same question regardless of who we are and where we come from.

It is the riddle of life itself that begins with discomfort, which in turn creates the drive and impetus to seek relief. Discomfort is like an onion. By engaging with the discomfort of our ailing physical bodies, we soon encounter the pain in our hearts that comes from a feeling of separation, and so the journey back to our essence begins in earnest. We embark on a journey of small revelations that gradually help us expand into greater and greater versions of ourselves until we experience one-ness with life, and that one-ness is yoga. But like any quest, the journey involves courage and strength because it is risky. The rewards are great but are we ready for the perils that lie ahead? Many have trod the path before us and we should take heed. Pay attention to the countless warriors who have moved through the dark and the light and left a trail of clues and maps to help us too.

The ancient system of *Āyurveda* is one such map that came into my path and infinitely expanded my horizon of understanding. It is the sister of yoga, as old and as profound. *Āyurveda* means 'Knowledge of Life' so it is much more than just traditional medicine. *Āyurveda* first concerns itself with what any mother would be concerned with: your health. She wants to care for you with all her wisdom. She goes to great pains to make sure you eat, sleep and exercise properly. She wants you to be happy and healthy enough to embark on your hero's journey but then she waves you goodbye as you approach the pathway of yoga. You need to be strong for the path and she has prepared you well. As David Frawley once said: 'Where *Āyurveda* ends, Yoga begins.'[1]

Āyurveda's great wisdom has made my road smoother and kinder and I want to share it with you. I want you to welcome its wisdom into your heart so that you can go on to share it with your students and make their journey more demulcent. It doesn't have to be that hard. There is no great urgency. Take your time. Take a deep breath and relax. Effort should be joyful and arise from within. Build a good foundation with *Āyurveda* first and you will be stronger. A strong you will be a stable foundation for your students too. Let me take you on this journey for a while, and then I will let you go ahead and discover the rest on your own.

Prakṛti: as nature intended

Mirror mirror...

When we meet ourselves for the first time as adults, we make all sorts of judgements based on what we know about life. Our assessment is largely based on social conditioning, which places us on a hierarchical merry-go-round of validity. Are we attractive? Do we have the right body shape? Is our personality acceptable? Are we likeable? This powerful undercurrent of anxiety is based on our survival drives that control so many aspects of our behaviour.

If we looked in the mirror with an *Āyurvedic* lens, however, we would see ourselves more clearly and celebrate what we see as a miracle. We are all unique and a wonderful expression of life that was created at a particular moment in time and space. We are an expression of everything that was born in that moment of time and there is nothing wrong with us. I repeat. There is nothing wrong with you and me! We are all life in progress, because Mother Nature *is* life in progress. We are evolving all the time in a spiral of highs and lows and ups and downs because we are an expression of the ebb and flow of life. Mother Nature or *prakṛti* is designed to be diverse, not uniform. We were not all meant to be the same! Diversity is built into the DNA of life.

Those differences are expressed in the way we look, as well as the way we think and feel. We have so many different ways of characterising people, because we are complicated. One of the great gifts of *Āyurveda* is in its simplicity. From an *Āyurvedic* perspective, we are all expressions of the interaction of the five Great Elements (*Panchamahabhutas*): Earth, Water, Fire, Air and Space. The physical traits, personality tendencies and disease tendencies can be expressed in innumerable yet predictable ways, and finding the right formula for a happy and healthy life is a worthwhile challenge.

Despite this complexity, there are, however, some common patterns that emerge that most of us share. The most common patterns help to fulfil the functions of life but as with everything in Mother Nature, the patterns are unstable and prone to corruption. In *Āyurveda,* these common functional patterns are known as *doṣas*. The word *doṣa* actually means 'prone to fault' because of its inherent impermanence. The three *doṣas* are as follows.

The three doṣas

Vata (Wind) is a functional entity that is made up of the elements of air and space. Its primary functions are *movement* and *communication*. Its home or seat is in the colon and it controls the nervous system, hollow organs, bones, kidneys, mind and senses. It has a resonance with touch and an affinity with the ears. Its waste product is gas. Its essence is *prāṇa*, which is the intelligent, electromagnetic, animating force of the body.

Pitta (that which cooks) is the functional entity driven by fire and water. Its primary functions are *digestion* and *transformation*. Its home or seat is in the small intestines and it controls the blood, liver and other digestive organs. Its waste product is *acid*. It resonates with the sense of sight and has an affinity with the eyes. Its essence is *tejas*, which is the inner radiance of the body that is expressed in the light in people's eyes and the brightness of their skin.

Kapha (that which sticks) is the functional entity that uses earth and water to fulfil its primary function of *growth* and *lubrication*. The body has been described by many as a 'bag of water' and in this sense it describes the function of *kapha* very well. Its home or seat is in the stomach. It also controls the immunity, lubrication of the joints and other aspects of hydration, growth and repair of the body. Its waste product is *mucus*. It resonates with the sense of taste and has an affinity with the tongue. Its essence is *ojas*, which is the inner strength and vitality of the body that serves to protect and nourish it with love.

We are all driven by the three *doṣas* because that is what it is to be human, but the combination of elements that make up our nature can vary. Our unique, personal constitution is called *prakṛti*. This word comes from the ancient Indian philosophical system of *Sāṃkhya*. It represents all that has taken or has the potential to take a unique physical form. In the *Āyurvedic* context, it also is used to represent the unique form of each individual.

Puruṣa: the great witness

Its polarising concept *puruṣa* represents the passive conscious awareness that pervades everything. It is the eye that sees through the seer of *prakṛti*, the drummer that beats the drums of *prakṛti* and the true taster of the food of *prakṛti*. It is Consciousness that makes a contract with its material counterpart to experience something of life from a very specific, limited perspective. Form is intrinsically limiting because it cannot be everything. It can only be one thing at a time, to the exclusion of everything else. A cat cannot be a dog at the same time, so to experience the life of a cat, Consciousness makes a commitment to that form.

These rather lofty concepts are an important preamble to understanding why *Āyurveda* and yoga are important to use together. Sharing or teaching yoga is a gift. Practising yoga is the gift you give yourself every day by paying homage to your Higher Self (*puruṣa*) through your body and mind preferences (*prakṛti*).

Let's go back to the beginning. When you look in the mirror, who is looking? When you decide if you are good enough, attractive enough, likeable enough, who is judging? It is neither your *prakṛti* nor *puruṣa*! It is a fear-based mechanism that kicks in that is commonly called the Ego. The ancients call this *ahaṅkāra* or *asmitā* (I am-ness). *Ahaṅkāra* is a small aspect of *prakṛti* with a very specific job: to protect us and ensure our survival. We all know excessive self-judgement beyond a healthy self-regard is not an ideal way to think, so how do we stop it?

The first thing to do is remind yourself of the following.

- You are free. You are only shackled by your thoughts and your limiting beliefs.

- Your limiting beliefs arise from an attachment to your separateness. Your separateness is experienced through identifying with your body and mind. Your body and mind are not you. They are only vehicles for *puruṣa* to experience the best version of you.

- The best version of you is a complex negotiation between the conditions of your life, your aspirations and beliefs in what is possible and the intentions your Higher Self or *puruṣa* ultimately has for you.

Āyurveda provides you with a map of what your *prakṛti* could be at its best. Yoga provides you with tools to help you sustain optimal health so that it becomes possible to achieve the best that you can become.

Vikṛti: your conditioned self

So far, we have considered your natural doṣic constitution (*prakṛti*), which arises from your parents, your time and place of birth and your karmic proclivities from past lives. Now we will discuss your current life situation, which may have thrown you out of balance and away from your natural self.

In an ideal world, we all hope to be able to express what is in our hearts and live the life of our dreams, but the realities of economics and socio-political conditions mean that most of us are having to live a life that does not fully support our nature. This so-called conditioned state is called *vikṛti* and, in life, everybody will recognise that there is an ongoing tension between who we are, the life we want to live and the opportunities available to us. We adapt to survive and, often, the adapted version of ourselves is so far away from who we are innately, that we get sick. This is not always a physical sickness. It more commonly feels like an uncomfortable piece of clothing that you feel obliged to wear that you get used to but never feels quite right. This is how we evolve. The discomfort drives us forwards and we move closer and closer to our own light with time and perseverance. But sometimes, we fall. We fall heavily and we are so off track that we need help to get back on our feet. That is where *Āyurveda* comes in. She is there to help you clear out the unwanted debris of an alienated *vikṛti* (the overly compromised conditions of your life) so that it can gradually come back in line with your *prakṛti* (your authentic self).

Dharma: the call of the wise

One of the greatest blessings in life is to be able to live out your Calling. It is so important that the Hindus have given it a special name. They call it *dharma*. Dharma means duty. In its highest sense, it means duty to the Self or the God in you. Some describe it as their mission or calling in life because they just know that that's what they are here to do. Most people do not have that much clarity and muddle along the best they can. Sustained yoga practice can really help to clarify your ideas yourself and help align you with your Higher Self so that you can experience the greater sense of meaning in life that comes from expressing or living out your true nature. This often makes life harder, not easier, because you realise that any path in life involves effort and commitment, but the ability to commit is much easier because it is supported by the conviction that you are doing the right thing for you.

If you are in the wrong job for too long, it can cause a sustained level of stress that can make you sick. In hard times, it is difficult to find work that suits one's temperament, so in many cases it would be a case of damage limitation, that is, making sure of everything that can be controlled, like food or sleep. The right job may not be an easy one, but it feels right because it matches well with your skills and personality. Try to find a job that is right for you. Not everyone is made to be a doctor or lawyer. This means finding your *dharma*, your right place in society. There is actually no perfect job. Every job, however glamorous it may appear to others, has its drudgery. Equally, every mundane job can also bring about a sense of accomplishment and fulfilment. Don't be afraid to change jobs until you find one that suits you. The wrong job can be a huge source of stress and unhappiness. Keep your eyes open and trust that life will create openings and opportunities for you to move into the kind of work that you should be in.

Kāma: the call of the wild

Kāma means desire. Everything in existence is born with desire. The primary desires revolve around survival: the desire for food, shelter, rest and procreation. The whole of society revolves around these primary desires, but beyond these we also have desires that are unique to us and are expressions of our *prakṛti*. It is really important to know what you want, to understand the feeling you are looking for in pursuit of it and to believe that you have a right to attain that feeling. Life will not always give you what you want but it will always give you what you expect. Most people are either very unspecific about what they want or don't believe they can really achieve it. Our desire for something is a hybrid of our conditioning (*vikṛti*) and our innate nature (*prakṛti*). It can only ever be that because our Conditioned Self acts as a filter through which our innate nature expresses itself. The 'out there' is the environment through which we find self-expression, so we have to negotiate with the terrain and try to find fulfilment from and through it.

Artha: the call for growth

Artha means wealth. Wealth is not just about money; it is our relationship with abundance. In general, nature tries its best to provide its creations with enough abundance to grow and thrive. It doesn't always succeed; however, it is worth bearing in mind that we are in the most abundant period in human history. There is less hunger and poverty now than ever before. It is not always possible to tap into the abundance of life if we are held back by debilitating beliefs about what we feel we are entitled to. It takes a lot of courage to trust the universe to provide for your needs. I believe that, as with many other aspects of these teachings, there has to be an interface point. Life can only meet us half way. We have to make the effort too, through our actions. If you don't want and act as though the world is abundant then it may pass you by. Overcoming the adversities of life takes a tremendous leap of faith for many. If you have been surrounded by poverty and desperation, it is near impossible to visualise any other kind of reality, which is why we sometimes need help from others. It is the duty of an abundant thinker to help and support those who have an impoverished vision. Nothing reinforces a poverty mindset more strongly than a desperate clinging to every penny that passes your way. Nothing cultivates an abundant mind better than to give some money (or anything) every day. Try it. You'll see.

Mokṣa: a divine calling

We seek to be full in all aspects of our lives. When our bellies are full, we seek to fill our hearts. When our hearts are full, we seek to fulfil our souls. *Āyurveda* teaches us how to nourish our bodies and minds properly with the right foods and medicines. Yoga teaches us how to fulfil the yearning of our souls. It teaches us how to find the divine from within so we feel complete.

The changing tides of prakṛti

All activity in life swings between a state of rest (*tamas*) and a state of movement (*rajas*). The best example of this is the difference between day and night. There is a natural place for both. When we are out of balance, the *guṇas*, *rajas* and *tamas* become disproportionate. We either become overactive (*rajas*) or torpid and lethargic (*tamas*). An overactive or rajasic mind is so turbulent that it is impossible to see things clearly, in the same way that it is not possible to see the bottom of a turbulent lake. A heavy, *tamasic* mind is so stagnant that it completely dulls perception, much like a polluted lake. Ideally, we are seeking a state of *sattva*, which is the third *guṇa*. *Sattva* represents the qualities of clarity, harmony and balance. Everything should be in its right place and in its right proportion.

The word *sattva* actually means 'mind' in *Āyurveda*, which suggests that the true nature of mind, when all things are equal, is that of a clear and high-functioning command centre that can control where attention goes and administer right action according to need. A *sattvic* mind is aware of its place in life and understands its power as well as its limitations. A *sattvic* mind is in touch with the wiser part of itself (*buddhi*) to make sure it is on track, as well as the more mundane aspect of itself that has to deal with the outside world (*manas*). Its wiser aspect (*buddhi*) is able to interface with *puruṣa* (Higher Self) so there is a strong sense of what is right or wrong when making choices in life. The best way to control *rajas* and *tamas* is to practise yoga, because yoga increases the quality of *sattva*. We feel more balanced and have greater clarity when making choices. We are less prone to the ravages of the mind and more likely to keep our *doṣas* in balance by managing our daily and seasonal habits.

Juggling balls

Life is intrinsically stressful because we constantly have to adapt to change. For many of us, life is like a juggling act and we are in a state of constant anxiety that any minute one of the balls will fall and then everything else will collapse. How well we adapt to change will determine how well we can stay in balance. Two people living similar lives may have very different capacity to adapt to life's challenges. This innate strength is also something an *Āyurvedic* practitioner might consider. However, *Āyurveda* repeatedly states that the aspects of life that follow this section need to be carefully managed if we want to maintain health and wellbeing.

It is commonly known that stress is the underlying cause of most illness but when we think of stress, we don't always consider the most obvious things. *Āyurveda* addresses the universal before it mentions the specifics.

DIET

This is a huge subject in itself, but the general rule is that what we eat should nourish us and not tax our system disproportionately. This rule applies to everyone but it all depends on how strong the *Agni* or Digestive Fire is. If you are unable to convert what you eat into healthy tissue, it will either become badly formed tissue that is holding toxins or has lost strength, or the food will remain in the system as a toxin that will eventually deposit itself in weak areas of the body and cause localised health problems. This undigested material is known as *āma*. This is the most important cause of all disease. Bad food or wrong food that is not digestible will become *āma* and cause ill health in the short or long term. What is food for one person may be poison for another. Get to know your gut's preferences. Pay attention to how you react to food and your gut will tell you! If it doesn't like it, it will usually produce mucus, gas or acid or cause mild inflammation and bloating. Don't suppress the symptoms with pharmaceutical drugs like antacids or indigestion tablets. Heed the signals and change your habits.

SLEEP

Are you getting enough sleep? *Vata* needs more sleep and *kapha* less but it usually works out the other way around because *vata* is light and *kapha* is heavy. You should feel rested when you wake up. Are you going to bed early enough? Many people in modern life stay awake too long watching TV. It is best to be in bed by 11pm and to get up around 6 or 7am. It is true that some people are more like larks and some are more like owls. I used to be an owl and trained myself to become a lark, so it is possible and you will be healthier for it. Is your bed comfortable and is it facing in the right direction? Most people living in small urban spaces have no choice on where they sleep. *Āyurveda* draws upon the wisdom of *vāstu śāstra*, the Indian equivalent of Feng Shui, and for optimal sleep it recommends the head facing any direction except north, which apparently is only for the dead!

RELATIONSHIPS

As with work, there are no perfect relationships because we are all a work in progress, trying our best to be with others who are also a work in progress. That said, there are people with whom you will naturally harmonise better than others in ways that are important to you. There is certainly wisdom in choosing to have people in your life that will support your values and choices. Commit to those people. Don't commit to people who emulate the behaviour of an unsupportive parent because it feels familiar. This mistake is made by many and causes a lot of stress in relationships, both romantic and platonic.

Āyurveda and yoga practice

How should we approach our yoga practice and how should we teach yoga to others?

As mentioned earlier, the purpose of yoga is to help students create a state of *sattva* so that they can manage their lives better and sustain prolonged inner harmony that can ultimately help them evolve spiritually. A state of *sattva* can be achieved with an intelligent approach to *āsana* that helps bring the unique arrangement of elements (Earth, Water, Fire, Air, Space) into balance so that *prāṇa*, *tejas* and *ojas* can be optimally expressed. One knows when this has happened because one feels light and energised (*prāṇa*), radiant and enthusiastic (*tejas*) and loving and blissful (*ojas*). There is an expanded sense of self and all is well with life and the world. This is why people do yoga. These are the feelings and sensations they are looking for. These experiences are not coincidental; they are there by design.

Please note, however, that these experiences don't last. No experience in the world of *prakṛti* lasts, because everything is in a state of flux. *Sattva* shifts to *rajas* shifts to *tamas*. The only thing you can rely on in the realm of *prakṛti* is change itself! You will have good and bad days and that's how yoga life, or indeed any life, is too. But the crucial thing is that the more *sattva* you generate, the easier it is to recreate the *sattvic* state when all things are equal. The hard knocks get softer and the bad days become mellow. The right yoga can end up being the biggest tool at our disposal for a life of less resistance to what is. We are all living out various micro-cycles in our lives and sometimes life just takes over. But regular yoga practice can act like a 'tortoise' to protect us from the worst storms so that we can live another day.

The qualities of the *doṣas*

Now we are ready to get very specific. What do I mean when I say that you should practise according to your nature? Can we box ourselves into a single *Āyurvedic* archetype?

Any system that tries to explain the mechanics of life will always fall short, however sophisticated it is, and *Āyurveda* is no exception. That's why it can only really be a guideline, a way of approaching practice, a consideration when making a self-assessment on how one is now (*vikṛti*) compared with how one has always been (*prakṛti*). To make an *Āyurvedic* assessment, we need certain tools. The first and most important thing to evaluate is how we are experiencing ourselves and whether that experience reflects a set of symptoms that suggest doṣic imbalance. The deeper aspects of an *Āyurvedic* assessment, like pulse, astrology and the tongue, are beyond the scope of this chapter, but there is still a lot we can glean by doing an objective appraisal of how we experience ourselves.

Self-assessment: riding the right wave

Understanding our natural place in the universe from an *Āyurvedic* perspective must include learning how to make an *Āyurvedic* self-assessment. Here is how you go about it:

HOW WE FEEL IN OUR BODY

The three doṣic body types are presented as follows:

Vata

Natural *vata* state	**Aggravated *vata***
The natural *vata* body is usually, slim, light, dry, either very tall or very short, with finer facial features. A *vata* body also likes to move fast, get things done quickly and has less endurance. A *vata* animal would be a hare or a mouse.	A *vata* aggravated body will have shifting pain, joint or lower back pain, dry skin, cold hands and feet restlessness and/or twitching. *Vata* is cold, dry and light, so *vata* aggravation also leads to constipation and back pain. Most people get *vata* aggravated at some point so should identify with this.
Note that a naturally *vata* body may not necessarily be *vata* aggravated. Moreover, someone with a *pitta* or *kapha* body may be also be *vata* aggravated.	

Pitta

Natural *pitta* state	**Aggravated *pitta***
A *pitta* body will commonly be medium build and height with good musculature, slightly oily skin and generally flexible, strong and athletic. A *pitta* animal would be a tiger.	A *pitta* aggravated body would feel overheated, sweaty and oily with skin problems and loose bowels. *Pitta* is hot and damp, so excessive heat and damp can also cause midnight insomnia.
A *pitta* person is not necessarily *pitta* aggravated and a *vata* or *kapha* type can also be *pitta* aggravated.	

Kapha

Natural *kapha* state	**Aggravated *kapha***
A *kapha* body is usually bigger and heavier, with big joints and lots of flesh. Facial features tend to be bigger and the general rhythm is slower. A typical *kapha* animal would be an elephant or cow.	A *kapha* aggravated body would feel heavy, congested and dull. There would be a lot of mucus in the chest and head and a feeling of torpidity. *Kapha* is damp and cold. Common *kapha* problems are chest problems and obesity.
A *kapha* person isn't necessarily *kapha* aggravated and a *vata* or *pitta* type can also be *kapha* aggravated.	

How we manage negative emotions

Vata	***Pitta***	***Kapha***
The prevailing state of mind for aggravated *vata* is fear and anxiety. Anyone who is *vata* aggravated will constantly feel the presence of one or the other.	For *pitta* it is anger and judgement. A *pitta* aggravating lifestyle will generate a lot of internal stress that expresses itself as anger towards, well, just about anyone and anything.	For *kapha*, it is depression and inertia. A *kapha* aggravated person can feel trapped inside themselves because of the sheer heaviness and density of their own being.

Of course, we can all experience a mixture of emotions in the course of a day, but if we really kept a diary of our state of mind, we would soon notice patterns that match with a particular *doṣa*.

THE QUALITY OF OUR DIGESTION AND BOWEL MOVEMENTS

My mentor, Vasant Lad, says that your bowel movement should be as smooth as the consistency of a banana. Anything else reflects what you are eating and your relationship with it.

If you are eating a lot of mucus-producing food and your body can't process it, you will see it in your bowel movement. It will be very sticky and heavy. This is typical of *kapha* aggravation or the presence of *āma* or undigested food.

If you eat a lot of fermented or spiced food, your bowel might feel hot and cause a burning sensation. This is typical of *pitta* aggravating food.

If you eat a lot of dry, cold food that your body can't process, your bowel movement may be very dry and difficult to release. This is typical of *vata* aggravation.

Putting it all together

Even gleaning this amount of information can go a long way to helping you decide what you need from your yoga *āsana* practice. To help make this assessment, the *Charaka Samhita*, a fourth-century seminal text on *Āyurveda*, has summarised the key qualities or *guṇas* related to the three *doṣas* so it's easier to make a match. Take a look at these key qualities and tick the ones that match your general constitution. You are allowed to tick two boxes in each row but not three. Add up your score at the bottom of each column to give you an indication of the key *doṣas* at play in your life. Bear in mind that how you are now may not be how you have always been. Try to assess your life as a whole so you get more of a sense of your underlying *prakṛti* than your current *vikṛti*, which is more temporary.

The qualities of the doṣas

Vata		*Pitta*		*Kapha*	
Cold (hands, feet, hates cold, stiffness of muscles)		Hot (body temperature, hot headed, balding, greying)		Cold (clammy hands, congestion, chesty)	
Light (body frame, bones, sleep)		Light (intolerant of bright light, sun, body frame)		Heavy (bones, body frame, weight, voice)	
Rough (skin, nails, hair, feet)		Oily (skin, faeces, intolerant of oily food)		Smooth (skin, organs, nature)	
Dry (skin, hair, tongue, colon)		Sharp (teeth, eyes, nose, chin, face, memory, mind)		Oily (skin, hair, faeces)	
Erratic (routines, habits, relationships)		Spreading (rashes, inflammation, ego)		Static (sitting, sleeping, doing nothing)	
Mobile (fast walking, talking, doing)		Sour (stomach acid, feelings)		Sticky (joints, faeces, relationship attachments)	
Astringent (increases vata, hoarse voice, uptight)		Liquid (loose stool, excess urine, sweat and thirst)		Sweet (nature, saliva, craving)	
Subtle (fearful, sensitive, insecure, twitchy)		Pungent (increases pitta, heartburn, anger, hate)		Slow (walk, talk, digestion, metabolism)	
Brownish/ black (dark complexion, dark eyes, dark tongue)		Bitter (taste in mouth, cynical)		Dense (fat, skin, hair, nails, faeces, body)	

		Fleshy smell (armpits, mouth, feet, socks)		Soft (features, nature, kindness, compassion)	
		Red (skin, cheeks, nose)		Hard (muscles, stubborn)	
		Yellow (eyes, skin, urine, faeces, āma)		Gross (obese, lacking insight)	
				Salty (water retention, increases kapha)	
				White (pale complexion, mucus, tongue, āma)	
Totals					

A doṣic approach to practice

Vata

A *vata* aggravated practitioner will try to bring qualities into their practice that will pacify the aggravated qualities of the *doṣa*. When I was young, I suffered terribly from *vata* aggravated back problems. I used to over-exercise and over-exert myself and caused a lot of damage. The quality of *vata* I most needed to pacify was movement. Even the yoga I used to practise was hurting me because it was too strong. When I finally realised this (by learning about *Āyurveda*) I adapted my practice and made it gentler and slower. Since that change, I have never been injured from yoga and have slowly managed to heal my back. Some might say that I might well have done that with intuition. One wouldn't need *Āyurveda* for that, just common sense. Yes, they would be right. *Āyurveda* is built on common sense and promotes the importance of authentic responses from the body and mind. But how many of us are really listening? Do we know how to listen?

The average *vata* aggravated student will be older with common *vata* complaints like joint pain, back pain, body pain, anxiety and restlessness.

A *vata* practice should be:

- gentle
- flowing
- nurturing
- smooth
- peaceful.

Particular areas of focus should be:

- joints
- hips
- lumbar spine and sacrum
- colon.

Pitta

A *pitta* aggravated practitioner will try to recognise what qualities are being aggravated. *Pitta* people are usually physically quite robust but are very prone to emotional upsets. If their practice is too strong and overheating, they will soon experience the anger and irritation all over again. In fact, a *pitta* aggravated person should always try to incorporate subtle practices into their daily routine as well. Mantra, *Yoga Nidrā*, meditation and *prāṇāyāma* are all very useful. The yoga world is full of *pitta* types because *pitta* people tend to be strong and flexible and like to use their bodies. *Pitta* people need to be very physical but the greater work lies in the psychological. A high-functioning *pitta* type will have great mental clarity. A low-functioning *pitta* type will be clouded with anger, frustration and undirected energy.

The average *pitta* aggravated student will be an adult with common *pitta* complaints like skin problems, heightened stress and an inability to trust and let go.

A *pitta* practice should be:

- diffusive
- steady
- surrendering
- cooling
- soft.

Particular areas of focus should be:

- mid-abdomen
- eyes
- thoracic spine
- mind.

Kapha

A *kapha* aggravated practitioner will try to avoid doing anything strenuous! They say that one should treat a *kapha* person like an enemy with the stick not the carrot. This is because there is so much stagnation that it is uncomfortable to do anything different or challenging. A shallow approach to this might be to make a *kapha* aggravated person do nothing but Sun Salutations, but this is wrong. The St Bernard dog, a typical *kapha* animal, gets arthritis and can be easily over-exercised. A healthy *kapha* person is one thing but a *kapha* aggravated person is another. The approach should be gentle initially to make sure the body is well warmed up, but once the momentum is built then a more dynamic approach can be adopted. Cardiovascular health is a key consideration with *kapha* types because they need to create inner combustion and encourage the channels to open and flow.

The average *kapha* aggravated student will usually be overweight, tired and swollen looking. They will commonly complain of fatigue, depression, lack of willpower and motivation and addictions.

A *kapha* practice should be:

- dynamic
- strong
- sustained
- moving
- mentally engaging.

Particular areas of focus should be:

- chest
- upper back and neck
- head
- heart and circulation
- joints.

Signs of improper practice

How do you know when your practice is not serving you as it should? If you are new to yoga, it may take a while to adjust to the new way of using your body, so a bit of pain and discomfort is almost impossible to avoid. This would be the same for any new physical activity even if you were a seasoned athlete. It doesn't mean you are doing the wrong practice. To make an accurate assessment, you need to give it a chance for a few months. If after a long period of practice you experience the issues listed below, or you initially feel good then after a few years start to experience them, then it's time to change it. Your practice should change with you. Our yoga should be like a dance. Life is our partner and we are moving and adapting to what our partner is doing. That is how the truly wise live and they live pain and disease free for a long time.

- Stiffness and tiredness (*vata*, *āma*).
- Inflamed joints and back pain (*pitta* and *vata*).
- Restlessness (*vata*).
- Anger and irritation (*pitta*).
- Heavy, lethargy and a lack of motivation (*kapha*).
- Ungrounded and unsettled (*vata*).
- Constipated (*vata*).

Āsana and the five *vāyus*

Āsana are essentially dynamic shapes that have an expansive quality to them and should involve:

- strengthening and stretching different areas of the body by moving into, holding and moving out of the shape
- opening out or gathering in different aspects of the body, which will help to regulate the *doṣas* that are seated, dominant or displaced and deposited in those areas
- moving the body in a series of directions once in the shape to enhance the flow of *vata* in those directions. *Vata* flows in five basic directions or flows (*vāyus*) in the body and is subdivided into the following.
    - *Vyāna vāyu* is the overall circulation of energy throughout the body. It is seated in the heart.

- *Prāṇa vāyu* is the *prāṇa* into the body from outside through the breath and drawn in through the nose where it nourishes the head before it flows down into the lungs.
- *Apāna vāyu* is the downward flow of energy that is seated in the colon and controls the hips, lumbar and lower body. It also controls all the functions of the pelvic region including micturition (urination), bowel movements and gas, menstruation and having babies!
- *Udāna vāyu* is the upward flow of energy that controls everything that naturally wants to come up and out like speech, exhalation and self-expression. It is seated in the throat but its origin is in the diaphragm.
- *Samāna vāyu* is the energy that controls the digestive tract. It makes sure that food and waste are sent, processed and redistributed appropriately. It is naturally seated in the digestive tract but its control centre is in the navel.

Here is an example of how some of these ideas could be applied to *āsana* practice.

Trikoṇāsana

- *Trikoṇāsana* strengthens and stretches the legs and feet.
- *Trikoṇāsana* expands out in a series of triangles through the arms and legs by either drawing them away from the hip and shoulder sockets (for the less supple) or pulling them in to secure the shape and make it more steady (very supple types). This will enhance *vyāna vāyu*. The spine is lengthening and rotating so energy is optimised downward through the tailbone and upwards towards the head as the spine lengthens in both directions.

- *Trikoṇāsana* opens up the front of the hip, which enables *prāṇa* to flow more harmoniously in that area. This means that the seat of *vata*, the colon, is acted upon so there is less chance of stagnation caused by blockage. It also opens the chest, enabling *prāṇa* to flow more freely and hence optimising the functioning of *kapha doṣa*, which is seated in the chest. The lengthening and rotating spine enhances proper flow of *vata*.

All *āsana* can be analysed in a similar way. It is really useful to approach *āsana* practice in this way because it refers to a broader, more holistic view of the body than just considering the action on muscles and bones. The ideal paradigm should be based on the *Panchakoshas* or Five Sheaths of the body.

Panchakoshas

- *Annamaya kośa*: The food sheath that makes up the physical body and is sustained by the food we eat. This is created by *kapha doṣa*, is nourished by *pitta doṣa* and organised by *vata dosa*.

- *Prāṇāyāma kośa*: The *pranic* or energy sheath that drives the physical body moves through a grid of invisible meridians or *nadis*. *Praṇa* can be controlled, manipulated or enhanced using *prāṇāyāma*, *mudrā*, *bandha* and the mind.

- *Manomaya kośa*: The mental sheath harbours our thoughts, desires and emotions. It is also known as our lower mind. It can be managed using mantra, yantra, sound, visualisation and other tantric techniques. Any meditation technique will help to gain control over the *manas*.

Most spiritual practices are concerned with the *manomaya kośa*.

- *Vijnanamaya kośa*: The wisdom sheath holds the sum total of our assessments and the beliefs and rationalisations that come from that. It supports the core beliefs that drive our day-to-day thoughts (*manas*). It is our intuition and our ability to discriminate between what is right and wrong for us. It is where the *buddhi* or wisdom mind is seated and is essential to develop for an easier navigation through the challenges of life.

- *Ānandamaya kośa*: This is the bliss sheath. Bliss and joy are innate in all of us and can arise at any moment without warning. It is an expression of the essence of life itself and largely gives us a reason to get up in the morning. The more yoga one does, the more *sattva* is increased and the possibility of accessing the bliss sheath at will increases. Everyone has experienced bliss in their lives and everyone spends their time trying to recapture it in any way they can. It is associated with the enlightened state but strictly speaking it is not this. The highest enlightened state no longer has an experiencer so there is no longer anyone there to experience the bliss. This may seem unfair but, in truth, *Āyurveda* warns against too much joy in life because it can cause exhaustion and lead to depression and loss of self completely. Bliss is part of the changing state of *prakṛti* and should be considered and enjoyed as such.

Getting started with teaching yoga with *Āyurvedic* themes

The best way to teach yoga with an *Āyurvedic* approach is one to one. This is because you get the chance to build a relationship with a student. You get to know their life habits, emotional tendencies and general doṣic patterns. This enables you to tailor make yoga classes that will suit their temperament and enable them to cultivate a truly productive relationship with their practice.

Working with groups

You can also teach yoga classes to groups using *Āyurvedic* themes. No one size fits all in yoga classes. Your adaptations will work for some and not for others. Everyone is different but those who resonate with the way you teach will keep coming to your classes.

Yoga and the seasons

The seasonal approach is an excellent way of sharing some *Ayurvedic* insights with your students.

HOT SUMMER

On a hot summery day, your students will recognise their relationship with heat. Some will like it and others will be oppressed by it. If you cultivate a class with lots of cooling practices, those who need to cool down, will appreciate it. Some examples of cooling practices might be: *Seethali*, *Seetkari*, left nostril breathing, relaxing poses with long holds (Yin yoga) and Shoulder Stand.

COLD WINTER

When it is cold, *vata* is potentially high in most people. A gentle warming practice is usually appreciated by most students. Include lots of simple joint mobility exercises, standing poses and *Ujjayi* breathing, which has a warming effect on the body. When it is very damp, *kapha* will also be increasing. Students with a lot of *kapha* energy will feel heavy and depressed. More heating practices, even in a heated room, will help clear blockage and stagnation and help *prāṇa* flow better.

SPRING

Kapha is usually melting at this time so students would benefit from a stronger practice that can help clear out the winter cobwebs. Sun Salutations and backbends will be of great benefit here.

AUTUMN

Autumn is a time when there is heat in the body from the summer and dryness is setting in. Heat-purging practices, like the cleansing practices of the *Shatkarmas,* are useful at this time. The *āsana* practice should not be too dynamic because too much overheating at this time can dry out the body further. A steady, rounded practice with lots of fluids and perhaps even a simple fasting regimen will be useful.

Agni Deepana: kindling the Agni

Apart from Patañjali's *Yoga Sūtras,* possibly the most studied text on yoga courses is the *Haṭha Yoga Pradīpikā* written by Swatmarama around the 14th century. It is a highly influential text that maps the key pathway that modern Hatha yoga is inspired by. It is one of four key texts[2] written around the same period that focus on a group of practices originally inspired by Buddhist Tantra, which was around much earlier. What came to be known as Hatha yoga is a selection of practices with a particular goal in mind. *Hatha* means *forceful* so there is a sense of creating a system that is enabling; a system where one can learn to take control of the body and mind in a very practical way. The system of Hatha yoga is loosely based on Patañjali's model but there are some crucial differences that make *Āyurveda* relevant.

Swatmarama recommends that before one can practise *prāṇāyāma,* the practitioner ensures all the *doṣas* are in balance first. To achieve this, he recommends the *Shatkarmas* or six cleansing practices. These include a variety of techniques including the familiar practices of *jala neti* (nasal douching) tongue scraping and *kapālabhāti.* The concept of *Agni* is also mentioned a great deal in relation to the *āsana.* Once *Āyurveda* is understood, it is evident that the *Shatkarmas* were directly inspired by *Āyurvedic* healing techniques. The *Haṭha Yoga Pradīpikā* is the first text I have come across that creates a clear and definable bridge between yoga and *Āyurveda.*

Agni means fire. It is mentioned in the *Rig Veda,* the oldest of the four *Vedas* and is arguably the oldest of all *Āyurvedic* concepts. I prefer to think of *Agni* as metabolic fire rather than just digestive fire, because it relates to metabolic activity at cellular level. Its seat is in the digestive tract because this is where food is transformed into energy and tissue. The mid-abdomen between the base of the sternum and the umbilicus is particularly important, because this is where *Agni* can be kindled and stored. In the *Haṭha Yoga Pradīpikā*, many of the key *āsana* and *prāṇāyāma* practices are considered to help kindle the *Agni*, and this is a useful starting point.

How do you know when *Agni* has been kindled? In *Āyurveda*, there are some key pointers. First, your appetite becomes very strong. This is considered to be an important sign of health in *Āyurveda*. Second, your bowel movement becomes regular and of good quality. Last, there is evidence of good-quality tissue formation that is reflected in the lustre of the skin and hair. This is a sign that the primary tissue known as *rasa* has been well-formed.

The *Haṭha Yoga Pradīpikā* lists the key practices that kindle the *Agni* and it is possible to create a course plan around some of these practices. Swatmarama mentions some key postures, like *Ardha Matsyendrasana* and *Mayurasana*. He also mentions *Agni Sura* and the various seated postures like *Siddhasana* and *Padmasana*. Teaching with an *Āyurvedic* approach should definitely include aspects of kindling *Agni*.

Other themes

WORKING WITH THE FIVE *VĀYUS* (*APĀNA, PRĀṆA, VYĀNA, SAMĀNA, UDĀNA*)

This is a very straightforward way of bridging yoga and *Āyurveda* in your teaching. Once you understand the movement of *vata*, you can integrate it into the way you teach the *āsana*. Arguably, all five of the *vāyus* are involved all the time. This is true, but you can isolate certain *vāyus* in certain groups for more focus, like *apāna* (downward flow) in standing poses, *udāna* (upward flow) in backbends, *vyāna* (digestive) in forward bends and prone backbends, *samāna* in twists and so on.

MARMA ZONES

These are sensitive areas around the body, similar to those used in acupuncture, that can be focused on with the breath and through stretch and palpation for a deeper experience of *pratyāhāra* and the release of localised tensions. The three key *marma* zones are the head, heart and the bladder region. *Marma* zones are 107 in number and it is worth doing workshops or courses on this fascinating subject if you would like to integrate them into your teaching.

Final thoughts

There are lots of ideas here and we have really only touched the surface. Take the time to read this again at least once to digest what has been said. You will get something different from it and it will help you to understand and integrate *Āyurveda* a little more. Imbibe the understanding first and then allow it to inspire the way you teach. Don't try to teach it before that integration has taken place; you will not be serving your students well.

In subjects of this kind, it is very easy to simplify things and give people the impression that everything can be explained away and put into boxes, but life isn't like that. It's complicated. Sometimes, people's symptoms can be complicated but the causes simple. Other times, the causes can be complicated and the solutions too. I have had very simple cases where clients experiencing a wide range of problems that appeared complicated managed to solve them overnight by simply drinking more water. Sometimes, there are lots of physical symptoms that shouldn't be there because everything is right, so it is likely the causes are emotional. This is the key challenge for an *Āyurvedic* practitioner. It is clinical detective work and it is very important to do this properly. Facile judgements have no place in medicine – natural or otherwise.

The *Āyurvedic* approach to yoga should be the same. Sometimes, a simple two-plus-two assessment equals four. We identify a *vata* problem, we change our practice and we start to feel better. Other times, we keep trying and still don't feel better. If you experience the latter, then get help. We can't see ourselves as well as others can. Let a trained eye work with you and give you options that you wouldn't have chosen for yourself. You will be surprised. We do not live in isolation and we were not designed to see the whole picture, because we are only an expression of part of it. When you are working with others, the greatest skill you can cultivate is *observation*. Watch carefully. Listen carefully. Don't jump to conclusions. People are complex, so don't be too quick to put them in *Āyurvedic* boxes. This was happening all the time during my training years. They say a little knowledge is a dangerous thing, and this is true for *Āyurveda*.

Equally, don't be afraid to try to help people. What works, works, and what doesn't, doesn't. You have shared what you know. That's all. Stay humble. Keep practising. Commit to your own growth and understanding and one day you will become a great source of help for others.

I wish you well on your yoga journey.

Further reading

Swami Satyananda, S. (1996). *Asana Pranayama Mudra Bandha* (3rd edition). Bihar: Bihar School of Yoga.

Lad, V. (2002) *Textbook of Ayurveda Fundamental Principles*. Albuquerque: The Ayurvedic Press.

Swami Muktibodhananda, S. (1993) *Hatha Yoga Pradīpikā* (2nd edition). Bihar: Bihar School of Yoga.

Notes

1 Frawley, D. (1999) *Yoga and Ayurveda*. Twin Lakes, WI: Lotus Press.

2 *Goraksha Samhita* (11–12th century written by Gorakshanath); *Gheraṇḍa Saṃhitā* (17–18th century written by Sage *Gheraṇḍa*); *Shiva Samhita* (17–18th century, author unknown).

— 11 —

Yoga Therapy

Training, Assessment and Practice

Lisa Kaley-Isley

Dedicated to Simon, my teacher on love, caring and dying well during the writing of this chapter.

Yoga foundation

Our ancient yoga forebears were curious observers of both the environment above and around them and human development. They wanted to know and understand everything and how it related, hence the naming of the oldest Indian religious texts, the *Vedas*, which translates as 'knowledge'. In the interrelated Indian sciences and philosophies to which we have access through the texts that survived, and the traditions that have been handed down from teacher to student, we can see the broad scope of their questioning and the depth of their comprehension. This curiosity to know and understand the individual characteristics of all things – from the smallest element to the complex web of relationships between them – is the fertile intellectual ground from which yoga developed.

The practices of yoga developed when the focus on this inquiry was directed towards understanding human nature in its changing (*prakṛti*) and unchanging aspects (*puruṣa*). The early seekers wanted to understand how human minds developed, experienced suffering and could be refined to experience the states of freedom (*mokṣa*) and enlightenment (*samādhi*) beyond suffering. They were curious about the meaning, purpose and correct course of action for human life so that humans could be free of suffering in this life and beyond life. Therefore, from its inception, yoga could be called therapeutic in intention, because the dual purpose was to reduce suffering and increase optional functioning. The founders of yoga concluded that identification with the changing self brings suffering, and identification with unchanging consciousness brings joy and freedom. To foster improved quality of life, and to prepare for inevitable death, yoga practices sought to decrease inner and outer conflict, to strengthen understanding, determination and steadiness in the face of challenge and to provide ways to experience joy and freedom beyond suffering through connection to the source of life while still in human form.

The early yogis observed that nothing exists or develops in isolation: everything does so in relationship. Hence, the root word for yoga is '*yug*', meaning, 'to yoke', for everything is joined and influenced by its relationships. When the connection between elements and parts is harmonious in a state of equilibrium, it is experientially different from when it is imbalanced or disharmonious. Imbalance and disharmony are seen as both the signs and stimulants of further discord and disorder. Conversely, actions that promote, establish and restore balance and harmony within the individual are indications of health and wellbeing.

The *Bhagavad Gītā*[1] and *Yoga Sūtras* of Patañjali[2] offer different paths and options on paths in order to achieve goodness of fit between the temperament and inclinations of the person and the practice.

Evolution and definition of yoga therapy

Yoga therapy in its modern form retains and employs:

- methods of observation and inquiry about the multidimensional nature of the human condition
- yoga philosophy and practices as a means to relieve suffering and to move beyond suffering
- selection and adaptation of yoga practices in response to each individual's temperament, condition and priorities.

We think of yoga therapy as new, because in the West it is coming into prominence after decades of yoga practice, but *yoga-cikitsā* (yoga therapy) is in many ways a return to a more traditional application of yoga than the group *āsana*-focused classes we have come to think of as yoga.

Over the millennia yoga has evolved and adapted to changing cultural conditions. In order to assimilate into modern culture, and draw benefit from both cultures, yoga therapy has incorporated Western healthcare standards and pedagogical techniques along with traditional Indian methods for training yoga therapists. Modern yoga therapy also utilises information sourced from allopathic (Western) medicine that advances knowledge and understanding of anatomy, physiology, medical conditions and, to some degree, psychological concepts. It also includes instruction in development and maintenance of therapeutic relationships consistent with Western standards for healthcare providers bearing the name of 'therapist'.

Yoga therapy, like yoga, is now taught, practised and studied around the globe. In recognition of this fact the International Association of Yoga Therapy (IAYT) was formed with the intention of honouring the contributions of the diverse schools and approaches and harnessing their input to distil training and practice standards for the current age. Over time IAYT has formulated a definition of yoga therapy, minimum educational standards for yoga therapist training programmes, accreditation procedures for training programmes, certification procedures for individual practitioners, a scope of practice, ethical standards and grievance procedures. As of this writing, individuals from 57 different countries are members of IAYT. Of all the members of IAYT, 81 per cent reside in the US, 8 per cent in Canada, 3 per cent in Australia, 2 per cent in the UK, 1 per cent in India and 6 per cent (271 individuals) in the rest of the world.[3]

In order to develop consensus from the practising yoga therapists, schools and associations worldwide, IAYT elicited definitions of yoga therapy from the providers and organisations. From the resulting data IAYT distilled and adopted this definition: 'Yoga therapy is the process of empowering individuals to progress toward improved health and wellbeing through the application of the teachings and practices of Yoga.'[4] Three key elements are highlighted in this definition. The first is that the focus in yoga therapy is not on teaching yoga *per se*, but rather on empowering students/clients to take responsibility for their own self-care and to provide guidance for self-practice. Experiences are provided in session, but the experience is intended to inspire and enable the student to reproduce the experience on their own. The second point is that while problems are identified and short-term goals may include reduction of accompanying symptoms of disorder, the long-term goals are enhancement of health and wellbeing. This clause also expresses the intention that yoga therapy does not claim to 'cure' disease, but rather assists in the healing process by improved coping and quality of life, relieving symptoms and fostering healthier functioning at all levels of being. Promoting health can serve a preventative role before disease arises, and it can promote healing by altering the conditions that may be sustaining disease. The third element succinctly asserts that yoga therapy draws on the vast repertoire of yoga in its entirety as its source for theory and practice.

IAYT subsequently crafted a professional *Scope of Practice* that operationalised what is included and specifically excluded from the remit.[5] The stated purpose of this process was to provide guidance for yoga therapists, potential yoga therapy clients, Western healthcare practitioners and all interested others who want to know what yoga therapy is and how it is practised. This guidance is useful in answering the questions that arise regarding similarities and differences between yoga teaching and yoga therapy. The 2014 edition of the IAYT *International Journal of Yoga Therapy* was specifically focused on exploring these questions in terms of the knowledge, skills and experience necessary to teach and be a therapist and the differing intentions of yoga students and clients. In the edition, Gary Kraftsow[6] asserts that yoga teacher training and teaching experience are essential foundational skills that are broadened and deepened during yoga therapy training. The accreditation standards for therapy programmes demand that they exceed the requirements for teacher training programmes in the depth and scope of material that must be taught and the level and type of supervised practice experience students must obtain in order to demonstrate competency. In addition, yoga therapy students learn crucial therapeutic skills that are generally not covered in teaching training, including establishing and maintaining therapeutic relationships, conducting interviews, yoga-based assessments and goal setting. Yoga therapy trainees learn how to apply the information gathered to develop practices that are personalised and adapted to the individual and to revise practices in response to changing needs and priorities. The curriculum includes development of skills to establish and maintain a therapeutic relationship over time and awareness of the ethical standards that are expected in the Western healthcare environment when the word 'therapy' is applied to the activity.

As the number of people practising yoga for health benefits has increased worldwide, government agencies have also become involved in the evaluation of yoga's potential efficacy to improve the health of their citizens. Some of the evaluation attempts were driven by concern that individuals could be harmed by untested approaches and some by curiosity to test the limits of what benefits yoga can help people achieve. A third influence was the rise in stress- and lifestyle-related disorders displacing infectious disease as leading causes of death in the developed world. Pathology-based allopathic approaches to counter disease have limited preventive capacity or long-term effectiveness to encourage people to initiate and maintain the lifelong changes in diet, exercise, attitude and behaviour that support health. Yoga, on the other hand, had ample anecdotal evidence to support its ability to foster these changes. In order to study the possible risks and benefits of complementary therapies, including yoga, the US established the Office of Alternative Medicine (OAM) in 1991. The office was upgraded to being the National Center for Complementary and Alternative Medicine (NCCAM) in 1998, and again changed in 2014 to become the National Center for Complementary and Integrative Health (NCCIH), reflecting fairly rapid changes in the state of the field. In each version, the centres provided funding for research and aggregated information from research to inform the public about the current status of evidence supporting use of different treatment modalities.

In the UK, concerns about public safety from treatments being provided by unregulated practitioners led to the formation of the Complementary and Natural Healthcare Council (CNHC). In conjunction with the British Council on Yoga Therapy (BCYT), the CNHC established minimum yoga therapy training programme standards, a code of ethics and a registry for yoga therapists who meet training requirements. The CNHC also established a mechanism for public complaint for complementary therapists.

Yoga therapy models and assessment

The practice of yoga therapy begins with gathering information from the client through interview and assessment. Assessment methods elicit information by various means so that multiple sources of data may be compared and integrated to form a more complete picture of the individual's functioning across the spheres. The purpose of assessment is to gather sufficient information to develop a personalised practice that will support the client in an integrated and efficient manner to progress towards the client's desired outcomes. During the process of assessment, a therapeutic relationship is established with the goal of empowering the client towards his/her own healing, growth and transformation.

Kośas

A key component of yoga therapy is the foundational premise that humans are multidimensional beings. The yoga model used to conceptualise and operationalise this tenet is the *pancha kośas* (the Five Sheaths). Most completely defined in the *Taittirīya Upaniṣad*,[7] the five *kośas* are different levels of interrelated being, which may be envisioned as Russian nesting dolls with each level encased in the other.

1. *Annamaya kośa* – the body made of food, includes all aspects of the physical body.
2. *Prāṇāyāma kośa* – the body made of vital energy (*prāṇa*), includes respiration and all the physiological systems that are regulated by the autonomic nervous system (ANS).
3. *Manomaya kośa* – the body made of thoughts, includes sensory information, memory, emotion, attitudes, beliefs, expectations, etc. conditioned by experience.
4. *Vijnanamaya kośa* – the body of discernment, includes the capacity for clarity, to make and act on choices (will and determination) and to hear and heed inner guidance (intuition, inner guru/teacher).
5. *Ānandamaya kośa* – the body made of bliss, includes awareness of the self beyond suffering and free from fear in an unchanging, illumined state of bliss (True Self).

Prior to the first session, it is common practice to ask clients to complete and return a written form eliciting demographic and preliminary health information. The questions asked on the form serve to inform the client about the scope of yoga therapy. By asking about each domain of the *kośas*, the client realises that yoga therapy is concerned with their whole being. This prepares both therapist and client for the initial interview. It provides the therapist with time to gather additional information about conditions with which s/he is less familiar, as well as to consider possible strategies of intervention. It prepares the client with information about what to expect in the interview and to decide what it is s/he would like to share in the initial session.

Annamaya kośa – *the physical body*

Yoga therapy with clients at the level of the *annamaya kośa* requires knowledge of anatomy and physiology, medical conditions and the biomechanics of *āsana*. It is helpful to have some knowledge about the allopathic and complementary interventions commonly used to treat them, including surgeries, physical manipulations, exercises, medications and dietary supplements that clients may also be using/have used. Knowledge of applied and experiential anatomy is important to ensure safe practice and to understand reasons for contraindications in the use of poses.

Assessment of functioning in the *annamaya kośa* interview includes relevant history, previous interventions, current conditions, presence of pain, activities that improve and worsen the condition and priorities. Throughout the interview the yoga therapist is observing how the client sits and moves to observe common habit patterns, potential asymmetries and compensation in response to pain or restriction in movement.

Assessment of the body and movement includes the following.

- Standing posture, usually in *Tāḍāsana* (Mountain Pose) to observe the alignment and symmetry/asymmetry of the muscles, joints, spine and head relative to each other.
- Range of movement (ROM) in joints, e.g. shoulder, knee, ankle, etc. in all directions the joint is intended to move and comparison with the opposite-side joint. Movement can be appropriate, restricted or overly lax/hypermobile. Both

restriction and hypermobility can give rise to pain, and pain can present in only certain portions of the ROM, so it is important to identify specifically where there is restriction and where there is pain-free movement.

- Directions of movement of the spine in flexion (forward bending), extension (backward bending), lateral extension and twisting to both sides to observe ROM, asymmetries and compensatory movement for pain and restriction.
- Movement in simple *āsana* to observe the quality, rate, coordination and alignment of movement in the whole body, coordination of breath and movement and ability to follow directions, perceive subtle sensations and make adjustments in response to them.
- Observation of seated, sleeping and walking positions may also be of benefit based on the presented complaints to observe common habit patterns.

Assessment of pain is a priority in yoga therapy. Experience of pain is often a motivating factor to seek help and make changes in life, and relieving pain can have a considerable effect on quality of life. Creating change when pain is acute is more straightforward than seeking to influence chronic pain, so early intervention before secondary complications arise is desirable. Assessing pain brings it into conscious awareness and invites self-reflection, which are necessary to identify habits, activities and times of day when pain is greater and worse. Assessment with a simple zero to ten scale, where zero equals no pain and ten is the worst pain a person has experienced, provides a simple metric to keep track of changing levels of intensity. Continuing to reassess pain throughout the session, and across sessions, provides information about how it waxes and wanes in response to rest and specific activities. If pain decreases over the course of the session, it suggests the intervention is helping and brings that into awareness for both therapist and client, providing feedback about what works and motivation to continue it. Whereas if pain increases across the session, or in home practice, it suggests that something is aggravating the condition. When there is pain, finding position(s), including *āsana*, in which the client can rest and move with no pain is the starting point for practice.

For musculoskeletal conditions, the selection of *āsana* is based on fostering symmetry, balance, alignment and appropriate ROM where there is injury, pain, restriction or the potential and desire to prevent them. These can take the form of replacing dysfunctional movement or resting positions with functional ones, increasing circulation, decreasing inflammation, strengthening what is weak and releasing chronic contraction. It is important to be aware of the whole body when choosing poses so that potential benefit from one action does not cause problems in another. For example, there are considerable benefits to mobilising the spine and coordinating breath with movement in cat/cow (*Chakravakasana*), but if the client has wrist pain, the benefits needs to be obtained either by choosing a different base from which do the pose, for example Seated Cat/Cow, supine wind-relieving pose (*Apanasana*) or an alternative hand position such as fists, forearms or wrists everted or elevated on a slanted block. Modification and adaption of the pose to the person are key principles in yoga therapy.

Doṣas

According to the observation of the ancients, all matter that has form is composed of the Five Elements: Earth, Water, Fire, Air and Ether. The Five Elements are combined into the three *doṣas*, which are always changing and going in and out of balance, influenced by lifestyle choices, age, the environment, seasons, etc. The *doṣas* influence the bodies of the first three *kośas*. The table below provides a brief overview of the ways the *doṣas* manifest.

The doṣas

	Elements	Physical qualities	Energy	Mind
Kapha	Earth and Water	Big bones and bodies, tend to have oily hair and skin, excess warmth and moisture, especially in lungs	Prone to being sedentary	In balance: steady and grounded Imbalance: depression
Pitta	Fire and Water	Strong muscles, fair skin, medium complexion, prone to redness and inflammation	Active and competitive	In balance: clarity and decisiveness Imbalance: angry and arrogant
Vata	Air and Ether	Thin and petite, tend to have dry skin and hair, poor circulation, cold hands and feet, wind/bloating in colon	Prone to being restless and hyperactive	In balance: creative and quick thinking Imbalance: fear and anxiety

The natural tendencies of the three *doṣas* provide a starting point to meet the client and direction about how to shift the client from imbalance to balance. For example, a client who is predominately a *vata doṣa* type may prefer a dynamic Vinyasa class to engage her mind and discharge restless energy. If she is healthy and well, the practice is a good match for her. However, if she is stressed and having trouble sleeping or digesting, in order to shift her towards balance, after meeting the client in her energetic preference, a yoga therapy practice would be designed to help her move towards a calmer state so she can regain the ability to rest and digest. In this way, *āsana* and sequencing are chosen to counteract natural tendencies of each *doṣa* to reduce excesses or increase deficiencies that may be contributing to imbalance, disease, or disorder.

Prāṇāyāma kośa and the prāṇa vāyu

Yoga therapy with clients at the level of the *prāṇāyāma kośa* requires assessment of *prāṇa* and the breath and understanding of the ANS and the physiological systems of the body. *Prāṇa* is said to move in five directions. The *pancha prāṇa vāyu* (five directions of movement of *prāṇa*) are:

1. *Apāna vāyu* – downward flow of energy, in the region of the pelvic floor, facilitates eliminative functions, exhale and letting go.
2. *Samāna vāyu* – equalising flow of energy, in the region of the abdomen, facilitates assimilation, digestion and metabolism.
3. *Prāṇa vāyu* – energising flow of energy, in the region of the head and heart, facilitates vitality.
4. *Udāna vāyu* – upward flow of energy, in the region of the throat, facilitates inspiration, inhalation and growth.
5. *Viyana vāyu* – distributing flow of energy, in the whole body, facilitates circulation, coordination of the *vāyus* and of the flow of energy throughout the body.

The respiratory system constantly adapts to the needs imposed upon it by the body and mind, and it also maintains habitual patterns of breathing. In order to identify habitual patterns and adjustments, it is necessary to observe breathing habits at multiple points, including during interview and during movement in different *āsana*, as well as formally while seated or lying down supine (on the back). Observation of the breath includes two principal components. First is the flow of the breath in its four potential parts: inhale, hold after inhale (retention), exhale and hold after exhale (suspension). It is informative to observe the relative balance in the duration of inhalation and exhalation, as well as any conscious or unconscious pauses or restrictions in the flow. Second, respiration requires the coordinated movement of the abdominal muscles, diaphragm, intercostal muscles between the ribs and the scalene and sternocleidomastoid muscles in the neck and shoulders. In the interaction of these parts, it is possible to observe if the client breathes more freely in the abdomen, ribs, chest or upper chest and throat, and what the coordination of the breath is like as it moves across these four areas. This reveals information about the vitality or deficiency of the *prāṇa vagus* and habitual patterns. Taking into account these factors, breath and *prāṇa* may be assessed by asking the client to:

- breathe naturally and observe the unguided flow of breath
- breathe into the four different areas of the body to observe their ability to influence the flow of *prāṇa* by virtue of attention and intention: abdomen (*apāna*), navel centre and ribs (*samāna*), chest (*prāṇa*), upper chest/collarbones (*udāna*) and coordinated integration and flow between the areas (*viyana*)
- sequentially place his/her hands on each of the four areas, or use other specific *mudrās* to increase attention and add sensory input, to see if this leads to any changes in capacity
- breathe into all four areas to identify any changes as a result of the previous steps.

To assess capacity to regulate the breath, ask the client to:

- count the length of inhalation and exhalation to determine if they are of equal duration
- ask the client, if the segments are unequal, to lengthen the shorter half so the inhale equals exhale. If that cannot be done without strain, ask the client to shorten the longer segment.

To assess breath coordinated with movement, ask the client to:

- do a simple movement such as lifting the arms over the head while inhaling and lowering them while exhaling. Ask the client to match the pace of the movement to the breath so that there is no movement without breath accompanying it. Observe the balance of inhale to exhale, fluidity of the flow of breath and movement and the degree of integration

- repeat this process with an *āsana* that requires greater coordination of movement such as lifting hips and arms in *Setu Bandhasana* (Bridge) or raising and lowering arms and legs in *Urdhva Prasarita Padasana*.

Limitations and obstructions in the flow of breath and *prāṇa* can negatively impact on vitality, in part because breathing patterns powerfully influence operation of the ANS. The ANS operates largely outside of conscious control, but it can be directly influenced by intentional regulation of the breath. The ANS is part of the peripheral nervous system, which coordinates activity between the brain and the organs of the body. It operates in two states that act in opposition: the sympathetic and parasympathetic nervous systems (SNS and PNS). The SNS, also known as the fight, flight or freeze system, turns on to support physical and mental activity, and it up regulates in response to fear that is present, imagined or remembered. Physical activity speeds metabolism of the neurotransmitters and hormones released by the SNS so moving in a yoga class can lead to feeling less stressed. Shifting out of SNS dominance turns on the PNS, also known as the rest and digest system. Yoga practice that includes activity and then transitions into rest in *Savasana* can further decrease stress and anxiety by turning on the calming half of the system.

The shift from SNS to PNS is aided by use of *āsana*, but it can also be accomplished by *prāṇāyāma*. Bringing equality to inhalation and exhalation tends to balance the ANS, whereas increasing the rate and duration of inhalation stimulates the SNS, and increasing rate and duration of exhale trigger the PNS. Breathing primarily in the upper chest is a sign and stimulant of SNS dominance, and breathing primarily in the abdomen shifts activity to the PNS. Respiratory disorders such as asthma, bronchitis, and chronic obstructive pulmonary disease

(COPD) where there is inflammation or damage to the lungs can result in compensatory use of accessory chest muscles, which increases SNS activation and further exacerbates their condition. People who are chronically stressed and anxious also tend to take shorter, more frequent breaths inflating primarily the upper chest, which both creates and maintains SNS over-activation. Observing the breathing habits of an individual, and their capacity to voluntarily create shifts in respiration location, duration and steadiness of flow, provides valuable information about their current condition and the places to start to empower change.

Prāṇāyāma techniques can be used to increase breath capacity, consciously shift the ratio between the duration of inhale and exhale, balance left and right nostril dominance, consciously employ suspensions of the breath following inhale (retention) or exhale (suspension) to build capacity and enhance the effects of inhale or exhale, forcefully clear the lungs, stimulate cooling in the throat or use sound to add a sensory feedback component and stimulate a mental attitude. *Prāṇāyāma* can be done seated and lying, and some techniques can be integrated in *āsana* practice to enhance the effects. The choice of practice depends on the capacity, needs and interests of the client. Determining what is needed, and what the client will do, is the discernment required in yoga therapy.

Manomaya kośa

Yoga therapy with clients at the level of the *manomaya kośa* includes assessment of ideas and attitudes, beliefs and expectations, fears and wishes, habitual behaviours, the play of emotions, levels of motivation, the capacity for acceptance, readiness to create and sustain change, distress tolerance, the ability to self-soothe and self-care and sources of strength and support. It does not require significant disclosure or time spent processing past events, as this is more appropriately the domain of psychotherapy and yoga therapy programmes do not generally provide sufficient training to prepare their students to be psychotherapists. It also does not include diagnosis of psychiatric conditions. However, gathering information about the functioning and contents of the mind relevant to present day circumstances is an essential part of the process. Information is gathered through direct inquiry, active listening and observing reactions across a variety of topics and situations.

Exploration of the realm of *manomaya kośa* moves many yoga teachers out of their comfort zone, and it certainly requires skills that are generally not taught in teacher training. In a group class, there is very limited verbal interaction between teacher and student and so this skill is not a focus of training. Discussion with students occurs either in the few minutes before or after class or by some arrangement outside of class. Even in private yoga sessions, many teachers lament that their students 'want to talk', while the teacher wants to move them into practice. Add in the intimacy of the questions posed above, in the privacy of a one-to-one meeting, and the reasons that training in establishing therapeutic relationships is needed becomes clear. The yoga therapist needs the ability to provide a safe space for the client to reveal what it is that s/he needs help with, and this necessarily entails a certain degree of both vulnerability and willingness to trust on the part of the client. Managing this relationship over time requires knowledge, skills, self-awareness and self-practice on the part of the therapist, as well as willingness to seek appropriate peer consultation and supervision as needed.

The *guṇas* are the forces at play in the mind, emotions and behaviour. Just as with the *doṣas*, everyone has aspects of all three *guṇas*, and each person has their personal combination of them that constitutes balance for him/her. Instability, excess and deficiency result when the *doṣas* and the *guṇas* shift in response to changing internal and external circumstances. One of the key intentions of yoga practice is to bring equanimity and stability to the *doṣas* and *guṇas*, and thereby to the first four *kośas*. The *ānandamaya kośa* is by its nature steady, but it is largely inaccessible unless the lower four *kośas* are stable.

Guṇas

The three forces of *prakṛti* (nature) are:

- *rajas* – energy, facilitates activity and change and fuels the passions of emotion, is the origin of life force
- *tamas* – matter, manifests as stability, heaviness, darkness, inertia and ignorance, is the origin of the body
- *sattva* – light, the subtlest form of energy, equanimity between the pull of opposite forces, draws to light, refinement and virtue.

Psychiatrist and Buddhist practitioner Daniel J. Siegel sagely observed that 'every symptom of every syndrome' in the Diagnostic and Statistical Manual (DSM-5) of mental health disorders 'could be re-envisioned as an example of chaos or rigidity... Whether it was innate in its origin, or caused by an overwhelming experience called trauma, having psychiatric suffering seemed to be manifested as chaos, rigidity, or both.'[8] Stated in yogic terms, mental health conditions result from an excess of either *rajas* or *tamas* that is either rigidly maintained or oscillates between the two states. This shows up in the physical and mental agitation of fear, stress, hyperactivity and anxiety with *rajas*, and feeling stuck, persistently sad, incapable and depressed with *tamas*. Some individuals are overly restrictive, such as people with anorexia, and others are overly impulsive, such as people with Attention Deficit Hyperactivity Disorder (ADHD). Individuals diagnosed with Bipolar Disorder flip between the two poles of mania and depression. Yoga practices designed to reduce excess *rajas* have the intention of calming, and those intended to reduce excess *tamas* are invigorating. As noted in the example in the *doṣas*, a practice that maintains imbalance may feel good for a period of time, but to create stability it needs to reduce excess without flipping to the other pole so that a middle ground balance of *sattvic* equanimity is achieved.

The vast repertoire of yoga practices can be utilised to help regulate energy, engage attention and inspire the mind towards greater health and wellbeing. The art of yoga therapy is choosing the elements and sequencing them to benefit and engage the specific individual in the moment and over time. Knowing what is important and inspiring to the person enables the yoga therapist to develop an integrated practice that yokes together the body, breath and mind with a personalised mental focus so the practice calls the person from their own inner wisdom towards a more harmonious and nurturing relationship with him/herself.

Meditation is the signature yoga practice for the mind, and yet for many people who practise yoga it feels inaccessible. In order to make use of this valuable tool, various practice elements are used efficiently to prepare the body and mind to be still, calm and inwardly focused. Keeping the mind engaged is assisted by providing the client with an object of attention that is pleasing to their particular mind. Foci of meditation can be *nada* (sound) of the breath or mantra, light or colour (external like a candle or internal and associated with a chakra), a chosen deity, yantra (geometric design expressing a mantra in visual form) or any other object that the mind can willingly and happily be absorbed in. The discipline of sustained practice for even short periods can increase self-awareness, distress tolerance, emotion regulation and the ability to hear the promptings of inner wisdom.

Vijnamaya kośa

Yoga therapy with clients at the level of the *vijnamaya kośa* involves assessment of the person's relationship to inner wisdom/teacher/intuition. This is elicited by questions and is noted in comments from the person that demonstrate self-reflection, self-awareness and whether or not the person has a clear sense about what s/he really needs to do to be happy and well. The ability to hear the inner voice of wisdom may be clear, confused or deeply concealed. Once it is heard, the person's relationship to the information may be in agreement or conflict. For example, when a person feels strongly that her path is art school, but her parents and teachers encourage her to prepare for business school. Or the person feels her sexual orientation is homosexual, but she does not want to face the feared negative social consequences in her family or community of that awareness. The inner knowing can put a person in conflict with him/herself or with important others in the environment. When there is conflict, this is harder to act on. The third step is whether or not the person is ready, willing and able to take action in line with the inner promptings. This is the level at which empowerment is needed to assist a person to take beneficial action on their own behalf. The yoga therapist needs to be attentive to the expressions and signs of the person's relationship with inner wisdom in order to offer well-matched strategies to foster empowerment while also problem solving to reduce or eliminate the obstacles that prevent it.

Vijnamaya kośa is strengthened by greater self-awareness, clarity and discernment (*viveka*). These are the qualities of wisdom (*dhi* and *buddhi*), providing the individual with greater capacity to make and sustain positive choices about how to respond, whether they are facing challenging circumstances, painful emotions or occasions for joy.

Ānandamaya kośa

Yoga therapy with clients at the level of the *ānandamaya kośa* requires assessment of what the person enjoys, loves and feels nourishes his/her spirit. It is important to know if the person in fact does experience any of these positive emotions, and if the conditions that inspire them are regularly integrated into daily life. Experiencing bliss and oneness with the absolute or True Self may be beyond the person's experience, but tastes of this can be experienced in loving and supportive relationships, in nature, in connection with a nurturing force greater than oneself, in the service of a meaningful cause, in moments of flow when there is complete absorption and in periods of creativity.

The yoga therapist uses this information to prompt regular doses of participation in whatever activities bring joy, meaning, purpose, freedom and fulfilment to life. The therapist may share with a client who is experiencing *anhedonia* (lack of pleasure) from depression, chronic illness or death, the yoga philosophy that s/he is not just the body or mind of the present condition and emotions, but rather a Self whose natural state is light, joyous and free of fear. When joyous and free is a long way from the person's current experience, finding anything that lifts their spirits is a start in moving in this direction.

Summary

Yoga therapy aligns with the traditional practice of yoga in which a teacher who knows a student well guides the individual to use particular practices that are chosen and adapted in response to her temperament, conditions, and priorities. The practices are chosen to be an efficient and effective means to facilitate the client's personal goals for healing, growth and transformation. A yoga therapist is a yoga teacher who has sufficient knowledge, skills and experience to act in this capacity for the benefit of the student.

Notes

1 Rutt, S. (2006) *An Ordinary Life Transformed: Lessons for Everyone from the Bhagavad Gītā*. Brookline, NH: Hobblebush Books.

2 Tigunait, P. R. (2014) *The Secret of the Yoga Sutra: Samadhi Pada.* Honesdale, PA: Himalayan International Institute of Yoga Science and Philosophy of the USA. Tigunait, P. R. (2017) *The Secret of the Yoga Sutra: Sadhana Pada.* Honesdale, PA: Himalayan International Institute of Yoga Science and Philosophy of the USA.

3 Kepner, J. (2017) Personal communication. (John Kepner is the Executive Director, International Association of Yoga Therapists.)

4 International Association of Yoga Therapists (2012) *Educational Standards for the Training of Yoga Therapists, Definition of Yoga Therapy.* Available at www.iayt.org/?page=AccredStds, accessed on 1 July 2017.

5 International Association of Yoga Therapists (2016) *Scope of Practice.* Available at http://c.ymcdn.com/sites/www.iayt.org/resource/resmgr/docs_certification/scopeofpractice/2016-09-01_IAYT_Scope_of_Pra.pdf, accessed on 1 July 2017.

6 Krafsow, G. (2014) 'The differences between yoga teacher training programs and yoga therapist training programs.' *International Journal of Yoga Therapy 24*, 15-16. Krafsow, G. (2014) 'Yoga therapy: the distinction between a yoga class and a yoga therapy session.' *International Journal of Yoga Therapy 24*, 17–18.

7 Easwaran, E. (1987) *The Upanishads.* Tomales, CA: Nilgiri Press. pp.142–146.

8 Siegel, D. J. (2017) *Mind: A Journey to the Heart of Being Human.* New York, NY: W. W. Norton and Co. pp. 77–78.

— 12 —

Building a Yoga Business

Katy Appleton and Natasha Moutran

When making the decision to start a business, or with any decision in life really, you have to start with the 'why'?

Why is it you would like to do whatever it is that you are setting out to offer? When you start with this question, everything else will fall into place and can flow from there. You have an anchor point from which to move, and you can keep coming back to this when you feel lost or confused with any choices or decisions along the way. Always come back to the why. With this in mind, it can be a great idea to write a mission statement to get you started.

Mission statement

A mission statement affirms the core purpose and goals for your business. It should clearly state your path and vision for your business, and will form the foundations from which you can build your business. This clarity will help align what you do in your business to its core values and create a compass point to which you can come back when making decisions. Your mission statement may change and evolve during your journey, which is totally normal and healthy, so feel free to update it as you go, coming back to it regularly and keeping it true and relevant.

Within your mission statement you can explore and go deeper into your reasons and purpose *behind* your intentions within your business. So, for example, instead of setting the intention of 'I want to teach yoga classes to elderly communities', you may state that you wish to 'bring joy to elderly communities through movement and breath, helping them stay mobile, connected and embodied' instead. This is a much more wholesome and productive approach to starting a business and will allow you to stay deeply connected to the roots of why you are doing this.

Take a moment to consider the answer to some of these questions in order to begin to explore your *why* behind starting your business.

- Why do you want to teach yoga?
- Or why do you want to open a studio (or replace this with your own business idea)?
- What inspires you to do this?
- What is it that you really want to share with the world?
- What motivates you to do this?
- What would you like to see change/see more of in this world?

These answers will form a springboard to begin writing your mission statement.

Whatever it is that you're deciding to move into, whether it be teaching classes, setting up a studio or perhaps you already have a business and are looking to change it up, a mission statement is a great way get real clarity. Your mission statement can be simple and short or may be more detailed and specific – anything is welcome as long as it is authentic and true, declaring your deeper desire in what you wish to do.

Feel free to take your time to mindfully write this now. Close your eyes, breathe and go inward to really connect to the true purpose. When you feel ready to begin you can start to put pen to paper. Keep going back to it and adjusting it until you feel that it really brings across your message.

Once this is done you can start to go about deciding *what* exactly you want to do with a more detailed plan or, alternatively, how you can look at what you already do in a fresh perspective.

Choosing the right business for you

One of the first decisions to make when choosing to start a yoga business is *what* your business is going to be. This may seem obvious, but there are so many options out there and the clearer you are from the start, the easier it is to move forward in your chosen direction.

When starting your yoga business there are many ways in which you can navigate and apply your teacher training certification into a career or part-time work. The options are endless in terms of ways to develop and grow yourself and your business, and we will only touch upon some of these in this chapter.

You could choose to be a yoga teacher in studios, in which case your business is fairly simple and straightforward. You may, however, choose to grow it into something far bigger than this, either with a more niche approach or with the intention of developing it into something far greater than just yourself as a single teaching entity.

There are a few questions that are important to consider when making this decision.

Grab a pen and paper, take a moment to close your eyes, breathe, centre yourself and when you feel ready you can begin to jot down some ideas and answers.

- Where would you ideally wish to work?
- Who would be your ideal student or target market? Try to be as specific as possible here and really picture your dream client. What do they look like? Where do they spend their free time? How old are they?

- Do you want to work for yourself or employ others to work within your business?
- How many hours do you wish to put into your yoga business?
- When do you want to work, ideally?

These answers will offer insight into what your options are for growing your business. For example, if you plan on keeping a full-time job and want to teach yoga on the side, then you must be realistic in terms of what you can offer with your time and energy, while maintaining enthusiasm and love for what you do and avoiding burnout.

The opportunities are endless within the yoga industry, or in applying a yoga teacher training to a career, so we are going to focus on just a few in this chapter.

The two potential business ideas that we are going to look into are:

- setting up your own yoga classes
- setting up your own yoga teacher trainings.

Starting your yoga classes

When setting up your own yoga classes there are a few things to consider right from the start, for example your venue – where are you going to teach?

Teaching in a studio

You may choose to start teaching classes in a studio that is already up and running. If so, you would ideally want to work towards boosting your class within that studio. It is important to build a good working relationship with the studio and to find a way to work with it so that both parties are happy. With many studios, teachers are paid an extra fee per head, so it could be beneficial to help boost the numbers in your class to increase your income while also growing both the studio's and your own student community. This will also bring you more regular students who could potentially stay with you on your teaching journey and could eventually support you by attending workshops or retreats that you might chose to run in the future.

Setting up your own classes

The other option is to start your own classes in your own venue, such as a local hall, school, church and so on. There are endless options for this and it is worth doing your research to find a well-priced venue in the area you wish to teach.

Here are a few things to consider when searching for a venue.

- Check the local transport connections and accessibility.
- Look at what facilities are available. Is there is a toilet or changing room?
- Can it provide storage space for your mats and props? This can be very useful, as carrying everything to and from classes can be a real challenge; negotiating a small storage cupboard with your hire is a real bonus.
- The temperature in the room might be something to note, as you want to make sure your students are comfortable and warm enough.
- Check the noise within the venue and from outside – what else is going on around you? Will other people be in the building and if so what are they doing?

Whether you choose to set up your own classes or teach in a studio, you need to attract students to your classes and let people know about your business.

A good way to do this is to flyer drop in the local area. Designing a simple flyer with the information needed can be easy and very cost effective. You can design something yourself and even print them at home to really keep your costs down. Handing out flyers is time consuming but instant, effective and well worth your time. Walk around your local area and leave them in local cafés, shops, businesses and clinics; just be sure to check with the staff first. You could also stand outside your local station for example, handing out flyers to commuters before and after work.

When appleyoga started back in 1998, this was the approach that got it going. It took time and effort, but it set the foundations for the business and was a brilliant starting place. The business is now in a very different place in regards to its development; however, these initial years were vital for getting students into the classes, gaining experience as a teacher and doing the legwork to be able to one day build the business to what it is today. There were no shortcuts taken, and it really has been built gradually over time, with persistence and hard work, which we can't recommend enough.

Consider who your target market is and where these people would spend their time or where you would catch their attention, and then focus your time there. This will also get you out and talking to people in and around the community you are going to teach in, so take this opportunity to introduce yourself and start to build a connection with not only other businesses, but maybe even potential students too.

Before starting up your own classes, research the competition in your local area. Are there any other yoga classes being taught near where you plan to run or are already running your classes? If so, who is teaching them and when? What style of classes are they? Take note of what is already on offer and see where there is a gap that you might be able to fill instead of going into direct competition with someone who perhaps is already well established in the area. You could choose to offer a different style class or run them at different times, so you begin to draw in a different clientele to the existing classes. It can be a nice idea to build relationships with the other teachers in your area so that you can work together and support each other's businesses, maybe even complementing each other's classes by offering diversity between yourselves.

Building a business relationship can also be beneficial with groups, such as the National Childbirth Trust (NCT) or an equivalent if you were choosing to teach pregnancy yoga, for example. Running classes in the same venue or offering a discount to these particular groups would be a clever way to tap into your exact target market and ideal student.

When running local classes, it is highly recommended that you build relationships with other local businesses. Find out who is working in your area and contact your local osteopath or physiotherapist for example, and offer them a free session to get an idea of what you do. This can then lead to you recommending each other and maybe them passing out flyers on your behalf and helping promote your classes. Offering free classes is a really effective way of building a good network and starting the chain of word-of-mouth recommendations.

You need to put in the effort and time to building and nurturing your business relationships and partnerships in order to see the benefits, but if you commit to this it will absolutely pay off for your business. These relationships can also work on other levels in regards to supporting your students. As a business, you must know where your skill set begins and ends and when it makes more sense to pass your student on to someone else, such as a body worker or therapist. Having a list of professionals who you can personally recommend is highly advisable.

New teachers

If you're a new teacher just starting out fresh from your training, you need get out there and teach. The more you teach, the more you will hone your skills, and people will start to follow you. Get out and teach what you know, be authentic and the right students will come. You can start by getting on cover lists at studios or covering teachers you know, and then let it build from there. It is important to keep studying; just one teacher training is not enough. In order to be a highly skilled teacher you must keep up-shifting, so you can stay on the pulse to meet people's needs. You may not need that so much if you're in a small community; however, if you have a lot of competition in your area then you need to keep building on your skill set to be able to offer a good standard of teaching that can stand out from the crowd.

Pricing

I'm sure many of you would agree that most of us choose the path of teaching yoga for the love of it and not really for the money; however, in order to have a successful business and be able to live off this career and life choice, most people will need an income. It is important to do your research in the areas in which you wish to teach and see what the going rates are. Don't undervalue yourself or your service, but be sure not to overcharge. There is a great karmic exchange that occurs in being paid to offer a service, so make sure you are charging an amount that feels comfortable for both yourself and your students.

As a yoga teacher in any capacity, you have spent money on a teacher training or maybe even several trainings, so it's important to keep a sense of value in yourself and what you offer but not to be so expensive that people can't actually afford you. You are now a part of a wider community of teachers in your city or area, and together we must uphold a sense of worth and value in what we do. Charging a similar amount to each other, and not setting rates way under or way over another teacher, helps to keep the balance and integrity of the yoga-teaching community.

That being said, it is worth taking into consideration your target audience for your business, as this will have an implication for the rates you offer. For example, if you are offering a luxury, high-end service, your prices would reflect this in comparison to, let's say, a small beginners' course being run in a local town hall on the outskirts of the city.

Setting up a yoga teacher training

Do you want to train people to teach yoga? If so, why?

Take a moment to reflect on your initial mission statement, and if this is your chosen path for your business then take your time to write another mission statement specifically aimed at this goal, connecting to your highest purpose inside your training.

Taking the step to start a teacher training can be very rewarding; however, it must be said that it will take a lot of your time, energy and effort. From creating the training, to writing the manual, to accrediting the training, there is a lot of background work that must be done. This advancing in your career requires a deep knowledge of how to deliver and teach in order to train others, which is a real gear shift in one's skill set as a yoga teacher.

If you are considering setting up a teacher training, you want to make sure you do your homework and take your time to develop a thorough and comprehensive training. Your training should be of the highest value in what you offer as a teacher, not only to share your knowledge and experience with others, but also to inspire them as teachers. It is a real honour to be a teacher trainer, and it is a position that shouldn't be taken lightly. It is your responsibility to qualify safe, educated and embodied teachers, and you want your training to represent this and your highest vision in the most eloquent and accessible way.

Once that huge volume of work is complete, which may take months or even years, then attracting teacher trainees is your next step. Your current students would be your first point of call as, if they have been loyal to you for a while, the chances are they would choose to study with you and deepen their yoga practice and knowledge with you. After that, you may then need to branch out into advertising and promoting yourself on a wider scale. There will be more on this later in this chapter.

A yoga training requires a good amount of promotion, and to do this you need to get your name or your business name out there. When you first have the idea of wanting to be a teacher trainee, right when you start working on the training, it is a good idea to start to build your platform and get access to different potential students so people get to know you and you can build a highly regarded reputation.

Get yourself out there in order to become known as a highly reputable teacher, beyond your immediate student network. This can be done by offering workshops, through online platforms or industry conferences or attending and teaching at industry shows, to name a few ways. There are so many ways to access potential students, so take your time to build a strategy for this and map out a timeline that feels possible in your world but also means you are regularly teaching and promoting yourself and your business.

If your aim is to run yoga trainings in a busy city, it is important to remember that the market can be fairly saturated. This is a great thing, as it means the world is getting more yoga teachers and therefore more yoga; however, this may mean that getting your training booked up could be more challenging, as there is vast competition out there. There are a lot of excellent trainings on offer, so you really need to know your stuff in order to stand out from the crowd. What you offer needs to be of great value and top, cutting-edge quality if you want your training business to work and last. So no winging it!

Our teacher trainings at appleyoga have very much been labours of love and have been changed, modified and adapted over the years. We are constantly looking at ways to improve the trainings and create an even better offering to our students. Through feedback from our students and our own reflections, we make sure that we are constantly reassessing to make sure that what is on offer is of the highest quality. If you choose to offer a teacher training, the work will need to be ongoing to stay on the pulse; the first offering may just be a starting point, so be prepared to do the work, respond to feedback, always look at ways to improve and adapt when necessary.

Finding and retaining your students

Once you've got your business off the ground and running, and you have students booking, then you want to make sure you retain them and keep them coming back. The way in which we show up as teachers and business owners will have a direct impact on this. Don't underestimate the importance of communication and building meaningful relationships inside of your work. Being a great teacher or a reputable business owner is one thing, but when you can do that with authenticity, integrity and a personable approach, students will stick around and come on your journey with you.

In the seat of a yoga teacher, or a yoga business owner, you want to make sure you don't just focus on the business side of things, but also remember that at the end of the day it is about what you are offering to your students. People want to be seen, and when you can honour them in this way, it will set the foundations for loyal and long-lasting clients.

There are many ways you can do this and sometimes the smallest touches can leave the most lasting impression. Being fully present at all times with your students is key. Meet people where they are at, engage with them and make them feel seen, heard and welcome in what you are offering. If you are teaching a class or training, for example, give a little time at the start to get to know them, their name and any injuries they may have and to introduce yourself properly. During the class, aim to adjust everyone verbally or manually, and try to speak their name at least once with praise or an up-shift. This is not only a great teaching skill, but also allows you to connect with your students and for them to feel that you really care, which they will appreciate and remember you for.

At the end of the practice, it can be nice to express your gratitude for their presence and for sharing their time with you in a meaningful way. Of course, as a teacher or business owner, it is important to keep healthy boundaries and not get too familiar with your students or clients. Maintain a professional stance in your interactions and hold yourself in that light at all times, so both parties are respected and held.

These human qualities can be really underestimated when discussing running a successful business but must not be overlooked, as it is vital to maintain that personal element if you want to build a lasting business with loyal and dedicated students. From our perspective at appleyoga, we can honestly say this has been key to growing the business. Building our community is one of the most important aspects of what we do and the response we get from students always confirms this intention, maintaining our connection with them.

Remember: 'Your vibe attracts tribe.' Stay true to yourself and let your true personality come through in all that you do, and you will see the right students for you come forwards.

Growing your business

If you have got to the stage of setting up your business and getting it off the ground, the next phase would be growing it, if that is part of your long-term business plan. It can be easy to get carried away and to jump to the next phase too quickly, and this is a common pitfall for many teachers and business owners. Take it step by step, building up a clientele before you go on to the next phase of your business development.

If you are a new yoga teacher, you need a good number of years of teaching before considering growing your business, for example running retreats or trainings, in order to get the bookings you would need. Let growing your business be a gradual process, building and shifting organically rather than being driven by force or want. Always be sure to check in to what the motivating factors are behind the desire to build on or change what you are currently doing. Be open to the signs and when you are ready to take the next step, it will become clear.

This might be accelerated if your learning curve has been quicker and you've been privy to receiving more information, education and experience in a shorter space of time, perhaps if you've worked closely with a mentor for example. There is no set time period. Everyone is different and will learn and grow at a different speed based on experience and time spent using and refining skills or the service they offer, so it is important to know when you feel ready to take the next steps and be honest with yourself when you are ready to do so.

Another great indicator that it is time to change or develop your business further is simply listening to the demand from your current students or clients. When you are in open communication with your clients, you can easily find out if they are interested in a workshop or retreat for example. When you can gauge this interest, you are in a positive position to offer it knowing that people are more likely to book. Don't underestimate asking your current students if they would be interested in something you have in mind before committing to it. However, it is important to know that just because they say they will go, this doesn't also mean they will, so manage your expectations with this.

Your business model may need the help of other people to run it, or perhaps you are working on growing your business or developing retreats or trainings for example. If that is the case, you may be in a position where you need some help in the running of the business. As long as you have the right person working with you, many hands make brilliant work. The question you have to ask yourself is: is that extra person helping bring in money?

Be sure that the cost of their support warrants the benefits of having them there. Do they cover that cost and more from the work they do?

Alternatively, it may be that their input into your business helps free up your time, which enables you to put your focus elsewhere. A good way of assessing this is looking at what your time is worth and whether you would earn more from hiring someone to help you, so that you can use your time more efficiently elsewhere. Or it could just be that you don't enjoy or have the skill set to do certain jobs, and therefore someone else's help would be a hugely beneficial addition to the successful growth and running of your business.

There are a few choices here that can help make this very possible in your business. You could, for example, hire someone on a freelance basis, or you may choose to employ someone permanently. Either way, you need to make sure it works for both parties involved and that you have a clear structure around the job. Write up a job description for them, even if it's for a freelancer, outlining their responsibilities, pay structure, time expected for them to commit and so on. Bringing people in to help run your business can really help you take a leap forwards and doesn't always have to be a big risk or commitment. This is especially the case with a freelancer, as there is a freedom around this working relationship and neither sides are tied in, allowing for an element of flexibility and exploration.

Branding

Branding is a huge area to consider when starting your yoga business. Whether your business is you as a yoga teacher, or something on a bigger scale, there are aspects of branding that it is worth considering and developing. Your brand is what will differentiate you from your competitors and communicate your company's identity to the world.

One of the differences between simply going out and teaching yoga and building an actual business around yoga is the brand you create. The brand that you build around your business directs the way in which people will associate with you and your company. You may choose for your brand to be a direct representation of who you are as a person and a teacher, or you may wish to create an entire identity based on what it is that you wish to offer through your business. If, for example, your chosen business is to teach corporate yoga, your branding may be very different from if you were, let's say, choosing to build a business teaching kids yoga. A good starting place is to consider how you want your brand to be seen by the outside world. What is the look, feel and voice you want express through your branding? This will include all your communication with your clients and should be a direct representation of what your main objective is – your mission statement.

The name that you want to work under is a good starting point for building your brand. This step should not be rushed, as it is important that it resonates with you and your mission statement and represents what you do clearly. You also want to take into consideration your ideal client and look at what names would best grab their attention and communicate what you do to them. Depending on what you are setting out to do, you may want the name to be professional, original or more symbolic, and for it to stand out.

You can, of course, work under your own name for your business, creating a nice look and brand around you as a teacher, although this could be limiting in the long run. Take a moment to consider your vision for the future of your business. Do you ever see it potentially growing or developing into something beyond just yourself? If so, using your own name for your brand could become restricting. If somewhere down the line you want to build from teaching classes to offering trainings, opening a school or studio and so on, then you may want to consider another name for your business that allows for this potential growth.

For appleyoga, this was easy, as it was based on the founder Katy Appleton's surname, and this worked well for any transitions and developments that then occurred in the business. When appleyoga was created, there was no set intention as to how big it was going to get or in what direction it was going to go; however, the foundations of offering yoga with a lens of speaking to all aspects of who we are as a human, body, mind and heart is what we hold in the highest regard when training students and therefore in our offerings within classes.

When you are deciding on a business name, be sure to check the name with Companies House (or the equivalent agency for registering companies in your country) and search for domain names to make sure it hasn't already been registered. If the domain name for the business is already taken, you may need to have a rethink. Allow yourself to get creative and come up with plenty of options, and then start to whittle it down to the few you are most drawn to. It might then be helpful to share these with some friends, family or peers and ask their opinions. It is amazing to see the response other people can have to a name, and it can be a very helpful way of seeing if your name is a good direct representation of the business you are building.

Once the name is decided, you can begin to develop the branding by creating a look and feel. You may choose to create a logo, which could be as simple as using a specific font, or it may have more of a design to it. If this is in your skill set, you could design something yourself, or if not you could reach out to someone you know or on social media and offer an exchange of yoga classes for a logo.

This is a great starting place, but developing the brand for your business is so much more than just the name and logo.

Have another read of your mission statement and ask yourself the following questions.

- How do you want to make people feel?
- What is your unique selling point?
- What is it that you can offer the world and how can you show it?

Be very clear in what you want to offer and let your branding– from the logo, to the website, to your social media – all be a reflection of this. Think of the colours, vibe and tone of voice that would best represent your business and its purpose in an authentic way, as well as appeal to your ideal client.

Everything that you do through your business can be a reminder not just of what you offer, but also of the lifestyle you are offering through it. Consider how you would want someone to feel when they leave your class and then see how best you can inspire and invoke that feeling in someone through your imaging, tone of voice and interaction with the outside world. Be authentic in all of your communication. When you allow for '*you*' to come out through your business in a natural and relevant way, the right student will be drawn to this. It can be an easy pitfall to feel the need to come across as perfect, or to be able to meet everyone's needs by offering everything possible, but often this doesn't work, as people will pick up on this. When you stay connected to yourself through all of your work and how you share your business with the world, the response will always be positive and will attract the right people to you.

Website

Once your branding (name, logo, look and feel) are all decided on, you can start to build your website. Your website could be wonderfully detailed and designed by a professional. However, a simple website can also serve its purpose here, keeping it simple and clear. You'll need all your relevant details on there, including what you offer, who you are and maybe even a reflection of your mission statement somewhere, giving a feeling of the 'why' behind what you do in order for people to connect to your core values as a business.

It's important to keep your website user friendly and accessible by making it easy for people to know where to find you or get in contact with you. You can add links to your social media on the website and maybe a sign-up link for your mailing list. You may choose to include some media, such as videos or images or have a blog; there are countless options depending on what you need. Whatever you decide to include on your website, it needs to feel relevant and connected to the business and to inspire you. It can be easy to get carried away with a website and want to include everything, but make sure that you are willing to put the work in to sustain it and be realistic with your time. If, for example, you want to add a blog, then know that you need to be diligent in updating this regularly and be consistent. The other option is to create a website that simply shares your information with no real need for regular time from you to update or add content to it.

Promotion and building a database

Any business needs to build up a good database of potential students and clients that you can get in contact with. This is how you can communicate with your students, letting them know what you have coming up, an offer you are running or your latest news, for example, which will eventually lead to bookings.

Gather emails from all of your students at any opportunity, always getting their permission to have their email address first. Whenever you teach, be sure to have a mailing sign-up sheet collecting students' information at the end of the practice, as well as adding people who get in touch via email. There are many free online newsletter databases out there, so you can collect them all in one place and stay in contact with them regularly, updating them on what you have going on.

This is a great starting point, but you also want potential students to be able to find you. You may be just what they are looking for, but if they can't find you then they will never even know you or your business exists.

Having an online presence these days is essential, both through your website and elsewhere on the internet. There are many websites with listings of teachers, trainings or retreats – whatever is relevant for you – so be sure to sign up to these. You will find a combination of free and paid listing websites, so opt for what works best with your budget. However, anywhere you can leave your details and people can access you is worth it. This can be time consuming, but the more places you leave your information, the better.

You also want to be able link back to your website wherever possible, as this will help with your search engine optimisation (SEO). Do check the terms and conditions of third-party websites, as some will have hidden booking fees or take commission even if it appears to be free to add a listing, although this can still sometimes be beneficial when starting out as it gets the students to you in the first place.

The trick to building up a database is to hook people in with something they can't resist. Offering free content is an excellent way of doing this, for example, offering a free five-day course when people sign up to your mailing list. This not only gains people's interest and gives them an incentive to sign up, but also offers a little taster of you and what you do, giving them more insight to you and potentially encouraging them to sign up for something else.

Another way of boosting bookings is to offer a promotion, such as a deal or discount on bulk bookings, or throw in something extra for free. There are many ways you can offer a promotion, depending on what you're wanting to encourage, for example if you'd like people to book a bulk of classes or pay for a whole training in one go. It can be a useful marketing tool and one that you can get creative with, using seasons or holidays as a theme for your promotions.

Getting your name out there is key to building and growing your business, and sometimes this requires getting out there and offering free classes. Once a month, aim to offer at least one free class or event that will get you meeting new students and networking. This could be teaching a class at a show or in a shop, or maybe working alongside another company, therefore gaining access to their clients and vice versa. Within saturated markets especially, people want to get a taster of what they are signing up for, especially if you are asking them to pay a significant amount of money for something, so allocating a little time each month to letting people meet you and get a feel for what you do will be very appealing and can do wonders for growing your business.

Social media

There are many ways to promote your business; however, in this digital era, it is hard to become widely known without engaging in social media or using some form of online marketing. If you choose not to use social media as a platform, that is absolutely fine and it is definitely possible to run your business without this. It is, after all, a very personal choice. If you do wish to engage in this medium and build your business in this way, it can be highly effective without being costly.

When using social media, you can either interact as yourself, making it a personal professional page, or on behalf of your business, speaking as the brand. Both of these can work very well, but will require a different voice and use of content.

Consider your social media channels as ways of interacting with your ideal client. It should be used not only to promote yourself or your business, or as a sales tool, but also to share actual content that can educate your followers. Let this be a way for you to share your knowledge with the world, maybe offering tips or nuggets of information or simply inspiring people in a way that is aligned to your mission statement.

It can be helpful to share some of your personal story too. People want to know who is behind the name, so sharing a bit of your own life can be a great way of drawing people in and sustaining their interest. Of course, it is important to honour your own ethics and know what you are willing to share and what you wish to keep private in your world. Do check in with this and be honest about what you are comfortable being public knowledge. Ideally, you want your content to be balanced between educational information, promoting and personal moments.

There are many different social platforms out there, all of which interact in a slightly different way and have a different focus. Instagram, for example, shares images with a caption, making it very visually focused and allowing you to build a moodboard of your brand that you share with the world. Using Instagram can be a great way of reaching a new audience, making use of popular hashtags in order to reach new followers and sharing interesting content. Think of this as a way of sharing a lifestyle and not just a way of promoting yourself.

Twitter is more focused on short phrases and needs more frequent posting in order to have an impact. Twitter newsfeeds are so fast flowing that ideally you'd need to be posting throughout the day to start to see the benefits. This particular social platform can be great for networking and engaging with your peers, mentors and other people in your industry.

Another social media platform that can be used to promote your business is Facebook. You could choose to set up a business page or profile in Facebook, and by sharing that with your friends you can start to build a following fairly quickly. It can be harder to gain new followers through Facebook without any cost, however, as it asks for a payment to promote posts and pages. This could be something to look into and try out, and it can work very well as you can really create a target audience for each post.

There are, of course, many others to consider and these are just a few examples, so do try out a few and then pick the ones that you find the easiest and most interesting for you. Keeping up with social media can be time consuming, so rather than trying to stay on top all the platforms, pick the few that you are most drawn to and dedicate your time and attention to building those. Remember that with any of these platforms, it is quality over quantity when it comes to posting, so take your time to create insightful posts to engage with your audience. Be consistent with your posts and keep them interesting.

The timing of your posts is also an important consideration, so think about when in the day your ideal client would most likely be on that particular platform. Commuting times are always good to engage with people, as well as lunchtimes or evenings. Once you build up these social platforms, scheduling your posts can be a very helpful tool. Set out some time at the beginning of the week to plan your social media for the whole week, creating a variety of content, and then schedule this for the week. Some social media platforms allow you to schedule directly on their app or website, and others may require an external website that can do this for you.

Whatever social media you choose to do or not do, enjoy the process and allow it to be a creative way of sharing who you are, what you do and your mission statement.

Finances, insurance and governing bodies

Running a business costs money. Of course, there are many ways to keep overhead costs to a minimum, but dependent on the business you are trying to build, it is guaranteed that there will be a cost involved in the start-up and running of this.

If you are setting out to be a yoga teacher on a freelance basis, such as teaching in studios or teaching private clients, the costs are small and can easily be covered by your income. You would be able to get away with a basic free website and your only overheads would be travel and possibly the odd promotional tool, such as flyers and your website. This is possible without a surplus of money and only minor outgoings.

If, however, you are looking to start or run a bigger business, it is safe to say that there will be far greater costs involved that need to be taken into consideration. When running a business, there are a few extra costs that you may need to take into consideration, such as corporate tax, staff, accounting advice, VAT costs, deposits on venues for retreats, travel, advertising and so on. These costs will depend on your particular business, but make sure you take all of these factors into consideration when constructing your business plan. Budget well and be ready to know you can afford to go ahead with your plan. Know what your overheads are going to be beforehand and what you need as an income to support this, as well as to earn the salary that you are aiming to be on. It is important to go into this in detail before even starting out, so you're not caught short down the line.

If your business model is on a larger scale, it is a good idea to seek professional advice to help develop a business plan and strategy, as well as seeking financial advice.

Insurance is a necessity in this industry, both as a yoga teacher and as a training school. Each of these requires a separate insurance, so be sure to be very specific with your insurance company about what it is that you need covered and have that all in place before pursuing any ideas. If you are planning on teaching abroad, be sure to check with your insurance company that you are covered to do so and whether there are any restrictions on this.

As a yoga teacher or yoga teaching school, you have the choice of being associated with a governing body. There are a few options in regards to which association you wish to be aligned to, so do your research to see what the benefits are of each, in order to make an informed decision. If you are looking to run teacher trainings then you will need to check the requirements, not just for yourself as an advanced teacher trainer but also the regulations set out for your training and school. These set guidelines are in place to keep the standards of yoga schools at a certain high level, help regulate the industry and make sure that only teachers of the highest quality are certified and teaching. This quality control helps elevate the standards of the whole yoga community and so must be respected and upheld in any yoga business.

Staying on top of things

A vital ingredient for running a successful business is being on top of the administrative side of things. As much as this may not be the most exciting part of being a business owner, it is essential and can't be overlooked. It must also be noted that having this side of things in order will free you up to enjoy the more inspiring elements more freely and with more presence. Being on top of paperwork will help create space, order and grounding, which are great foundations to build a business on. Start this healthy relationship with the administrative work from the get go and you'll find it easier to stay on top of it throughout your career.

Running a yoga business requires a lot more than simply teaching yoga classes. However, the admin does not have to take over your life, as this can easily start taking away from time offered to actual teaching or developing your work. The key is to work smarter, not harder, and have set boundaries around your approach to admin, such as emails and paperwork. Put aside a few hours a day, in one go or split into two parts, to do all your admin, commit to completing the essential jobs in that time and then walk away. Getting into this habit is a blessing in your working life as it can be easy to get stuck at your laptop.

It can be easy to get glued to a desk, creating more work than necessary, which is not a productive use of time. So allocating a set time schedule in your day or week to get admin and emails done can help you be far more efficient with your time. Plan your week in advance so you know when these time slots will be and then be sure to allow time for creativity, teaching and inspiration in order to make your business flow. Creating an auto response on your emails can support this work schedule and manage clients' expectations so that they know when to expect a reply from you.

Be online everyday, but be diligent about how long you spend on this and have a set cut-off time. You can then use that extra energy and put it elsewhere where it will be more productive. Don't give it all to the internet. Keeping your inspiration alive will also help avoid burnout, which is a common pitfall, not only for new teachers and business owners, but also for even the more experienced.

When it comes to running a yoga business, always stay true to your bigger purpose and highest vision. At times it will be hard, and you will meet challenges along the way, but know that these ups and downs are totally normal and come as part of this journey to make you grow and progress as a business. At times you will make mistakes, but as long as you can take the time to notice these, learn from them, and then move on, you will be on the right path for a successful business. Starting your own business can be incredibly scary, but know that as long as you stay on course and keep coming back to the why and staying connected to your mission statement, you will always be able to steer it back on track and make it work. Whatever happens, make sure you continue to love and enjoy what you do. Good luck!

— 13 —

Running a Yoga Retreat

Kate Walker

Teaching a yoga retreat sounds, on paper, like the best thing ever: being paid to go on holiday while being able to work more closely and consistently with students. What's not to love?

Slow down there, my friend! In order to run a successful retreat there are stages to be aware of, for your own sake as well as for the students'. In this chapter, we look at how to set up, run and follow up a retreat so it runs smoothly. I will share some questions to ask about yourself, as well as questions about the venue and the students, in order to clarify intention, manage expectations and ensure the whole experience runs smoothly.

I started teaching retreats roughly five years after I started teaching yoga. I was asked by a well-known company specialising in wellness and health retreats to come away with them to far-flung places and teach yoga on their weeks. I was so excited and honoured to be asked. I taught for them for a few years, which had its advantages: I went all over the world and didn't have to manage or sort anything myself. They even booked my flights for me. But it also had its disadvantages: they didn't pay particularly well; I found the client base to be more interested in losing weight on the weeks than practising yoga, so often felt I was teaching a stretch class as opposed to the more heart-based work I specialise in; I had to teach many classes each day from early in the morning until late in the evening, which was more than I was used to; I always had to share a room – sometimes even a bed – with two to four (albeit female) staff (the nutritionist, personal trainer, etc.).

I then taught yoga-only retreats for a few different companies, which was equally easy and low-maintenance for me, but, similarly, didn't pay particularly well and wasn't as satisfying as working with my regular students. Serious yoga students don't tend to go on a yoga retreat with a teacher they haven't met before, so there was often a lack of dedication to the student base.

After I had taught quite a few retreats through various companies, I realised I had my own student base who were interested in retreats with me, so I started teaching my own. The first retreat I taught was a weekend in Portugal. I taught the yoga, my husband did the cooking and my friend assisted during classes. I taught two classes a day to ten students. I found it exhilarating to have the time to go deeper with my students and to get paid well for doing so in a beautiful country. But I also found it completely exhausting. In just three days I was drained.

That was over a decade ago now, and since then I've learned how to protect myself from burnout and lead retreats that are nourishing for the students and also for myself. Retreats can be a wonderful experience, if planned carefully and thoroughly.

Step 1: Laying the foundation

What is a yoga retreat? A retreat is anything that takes the students away from their everyday life and gives them more time and space to practise. This can be a day, weekend, week or even longer. Most commonly, retreats last one week and are somewhere beautiful and relaxing so the student feels as if they are on holiday, as well as having extra time for their yoga. Go on some yoga retreats yourself, and note what works for you and what doesn't.

The first thing to consider is whether you do in fact want to host a retreat – sounds silly, I know, but are you responsible and organised? Do you embrace admin? Do you have a sufficient student base to attract enough paying clients to make it work financially? Does your insurance cover you to teach retreats? If admin isn't your thing, maybe getting someone to do the organising and emailing etc. for you is an option – they could be paid or given a free space on the retreat as compensation. If you don't have the student base, there are companies that host retreats that look for yoga teachers to come teach for them – it might be a nice option to get used to 'holding space' (something I'll talk about later) while you're still building your clientele. You might also join forces with another teacher and share the organising, marketing and teaching, but then be prepared to share the profits too.

Where do you want to go? There are benefits from staying local: a train or car ride is easier and cheaper for the attendee. A little further afield, a short flight with not much jetlag, can be a great option. A long-haul flight can be a real adventure, but adds cost to you and the student, and jetlag can be difficult to manage.

When you've decided where you want to go, it's time to look for a venue. Consider whether you want exclusive use of the venue, which is a luxury, as your group of yogis will be the only people at the venue during your retreat. This can often help the students let go and open up, as they feel unguarded and safe. Consider whether having exclusive use truly matters to you or your students; it will open up more options for locations if you don't commit to taking over the whole venue, as finding a venue that is the perfect size for your students – not too big and not too small – is tricky.

The three most important things to look for are:

- a big enough and appropriate yoga space
- enough beds/rooms for your group
- good communication from the venue and great customer service.

A big enough and appropriate yoga space

By 'appropriate yoga space' I mean is it big enough for the group? Does it have what you need? For example, if you teach Iyengar yoga, does it have props and/or ropes? You won't want to bring all the props with you. Will you have full use of it during the class times you plan, and what will happen with the space when you're not in class? (I once taught a retreat where the yoga space was used as a smoking lounge when we weren't in class.) Is it very exposed? (This might make the students self-conscious.) Is it just next to a road, disco or something loud and distracting? Photos might show a serene space, so it's a good idea to ask more specific questions. It's an even better idea to go see the venue before you hold your retreat there.

Enough beds/rooms for the group

You want to have enough options for students who want their own room and students who want to come with their partners or their friends. You need twin rooms, double rooms and single rooms. Are they en suite or do the students share a bathroom? It's a fine balance: you wouldn't want to hold a retreat in a venue with 600 rooms, which will feel vast and impersonal, or a venue with only five rooms, which will make it difficult to make a profit with so few students.

Good communication with the venue and great customer service

You want the venue to respond to your questions clearly and in a timely manner. Someone you deal with must speak your language. If something happens while you're hosting the retreat, you need to be able to ask for their advice and help. Trust your gut while dealing with them, too. I have dealt with some venues that have made me feel they were doing me a huge favour by letting me host there, which was a disaster as I (and the students) picked up on this during the whole week and felt as if we were a burden to them and they didn't want us there. Remember that you're bringing them good business (as long as you are clear, organised and easy to deal with yourself), and if it goes well you might host many retreats there in future, so it's beneficial to them to have you.

Even large companies struggle with setting prices. It's complicated and difficult. You have to be aware first of all of how much it will cost you: how much the venue will take, how much it will cost for you to get there and be there (travel, food, your own accommodation), how much you want to make as profit and so on. Research how much comparable retreats cost, and consider how much your student base will be willing to pay. For example, if you happen to teach a bunch of millionaires, you can probably host in a swanky place and charge a lot of money. For most of us, however, we teach normal people with normal incomes for whom a holiday is a big expense, so we must find a balance between charging too little so you don't break even and charging too much so no one can afford to sign up.

You might consider early-bird special offers to encourage people to book early. You might consider discounts if someone brings a friend. Usually, there are different price points you can offer, based on the luxury of the room chosen (venue dependent) or whether that person is sharing with three others or paying a single supplement to have their own room. Be aware that the venue will ask for a large deposit or even for you to pay in full upfront. This can be scary: it puts you at risk of being out of pocket if you don't get enough students to sign up.

Do your research on the venue; there are great sites online that serve as a platform for guest reviews, for example TripAdvisor. Guests post photos and write personal reviews based on their experience. This has proved invaluable to me in the past. Yet, as I mentioned earlier, ideally, go and see the venue yourself before you host there. Practise in the space, eat where the students will eat… Then you'll really know whether it will work or not.

Make sure you and the venue come to a clear agreement, in writing, about pricing. What happens if you book ten rooms and then end up only using six? What happens if you end up needing 12? What will they include in your package, i.e. what food is included per person? Do they organise transfers to or from the airport/station? What deposit do they require from you to hold the rooms and space for your retreat, and when will the balance be due? Keep all the agreements printed in a file, and take that file with you on the retreat so it's easily referenced if necessary.

Ready, steady, go!

When you've decided on the venue, booked the time and agreed the contract, it's time to think about marketing. Making flyers to give to your students is an easy way to spread the news – get some high-resolution photographs of the venue and of yourself to put on the flyers. Make sure the flyers contain just enough information so that what to expect is clear to those interested. Give flyers out in classes and leave some in local shops, gyms or studios (with prior permission).

Things to include on your flyer are:

- the date of the retreat
- who you are (assuming you're the teacher)
- where it'll be
- pricing (and what that includes, as well as what that doesn't include)
- a description of the retreat – how many classes a day, any other excursions or opportunities that are available (e.g. massage, scuba diving)
- how to get in contact with you/find out more (e.g. a website with further information and photographs) and/or book the retreat.

There are other ways to promote your retreat as well: have a newsletter you send out, use social media (Twitter, Facebook, Instagram) and perhaps promote on third-party websites (this might cost a small fee) that specialise in retreats. Most, if not all, of the students who come on the retreat will come because they want to work with you. Some will come just because the dates or the place appeal to them. Either group will hear about the retreat because of your efforts, so spread the word as much as you can.

It is hoped that these various methods of marketing will result in interest. Make yourself easy to find and readily available for questions and bookings. Note the questions that come in, as you might be able to form an FAQ section on your website to head off the most frequent questions before they are even asked. When someone wants to book, take a deposit. I have taken 30 per cent and 50 per cent deposits in the past, depending on the retreat. Clarify whether this is a non-refundable deposit or if there are any circumstances in which cancellation would be acceptable. For example, if someone cancels due to pregnancy, would the deposit be refunded or would you transfer them to a different retreat post-baby? If someone cancels three months before the retreat, are the rules different from if they cancel two days before? Explain when the balance will be due, and make sure you send out reminder emails in good time. Encourage students to have their own health and travel insurance. Once I had to cancel a retreat that was scheduled to take place in an Egyptian Red Sea resort following a political issue that resulted in all the UK flights being suspended to and from the destination. I refunded the students but could not refund them what they had spent on their own flights. This is when having their own travel insurance is important. Make the rules clear to avoid awkward situations in the future.

Communicate with the students when they book about who they are, what their expectations are and anything else you should be aware of, for example, medical conditions, dietary restrictions, yoga experience, injuries and medication taken. This will help you design your classes and know more about how to best serve the group. If your group becomes very large, consider bringing an assistant to help you during the classes so that the students are properly looked after. You might bring a massage therapist along to treat the guests (consider whether the massages are included in the price or, if they will cost extra, tell the students they can book massages for a supplementary fee). Make it known that you are not a tour operator (this is important for insurance reasons) so the students must book their own flights. You might consider getting the students to sign a waiver upon booking, acknowledging that they accept responsibility for their travel and health during the retreat.

Book your own travel in good time, establishing a 'recommended' flight or train so that most students end up on the same form of transport – this makes transport from the airport/station to the venue easier. It has worked well in the past to include transfers if the students take the recommended flights and to be able to arrange separate transfers (for an extra fee) if they decide to take a different flight. Often, the venue can help arrange a transfer coach for the students. You might decide to bring a romantic partner with you, which is fine (and nice for you as well as for them) as long as they add to the retreat rather than distract you and take you away from your students.

You may or may not decide to have a 'Plan B': i.e. an alternative venue if the one you've booked ends up being problematic, or an alternative teacher if you end up being sick or injured. I've never had a Plan B, but had to cancel a retreat once (as I mentioned earlier) because UK flights in and out of our destination were suspended over terrorism fears. If I had had an alternative venue in mind I would have been able to keep the retreat going and just change the location. I've never had to get a different teacher to teach – I've taught through injury, sickness and pregnancy. But once on a retreat I got sick and needed to take an afternoon off. Luckily, I usually offer an afternoon off at some point during the week for students to take excursions or rest, so all I had to do was change the day that applied to the day I was sick and the students didn't miss any class. This is why it's important to specify that schedules are 'subject to change'.

Nearly there...

So you've gathered your group and you've been paid the deposits and the balances: the time to go is nearly upon you. I recommend sending out an email to all the guests (use BCC for privacy) with reminders on what to bring (clothes, mosquito spray, sun cream or sweaters; do they need towels? Do they need their own yoga mat/props?) and an outline of what they'll be doing. It's always good to be overly clear rather than not clear enough. Remind the students of which method of transport they're taking, what will happen when they arrive and what to expect that first day/evening/night. If students are driving, send a PDF of driving directions. Students should know how to contact both you and the venue if something goes wrong. I have had students forget their passport, miss their flight and get lost in the airport: make sure they know what to do and who to contact if anything happens.

And we're off!

It is your choice about whether to arrive before the guests or with them. Avoid at all costs arriving after them. The benefit to arriving before them is that you can set up the yoga space, perhaps leave welcome notes with printed schedules on their beds, organise with the hotel any last minute things and be there when the students arrive to welcome them. The benefit to arriving with them is you'll be there to help make the transport easy. For example, if you're all on a recommended flight and then there's a two hour coach journey, the students might like to meet you at the airport and all take the coach together, rather than meeting you at the venue after the flight and coach journey. This decision partly depends on how much you trust the venue to set things up for you.

Know what you'll need during your time away – not only for yourself, but also bring things 'just in case', like a first aid kit. If you use music during your classes, bring portable speakers if the yoga space doesn't have a sound system. Ensure you have the props you'll want, any candles or incense or anything you like teaching with. I always travel with my little yoga quote book and some Tibetan bells. Ask the venue if there's a laundry service and if the cost is included. You will then need to pack accordingly: bringing enough yoga clothes for each and every class or using the laundry service and packing more sparingly.

We've arrived!

Little details to make the guests feel welcome go a long way. If the retreat is held somewhere hot, it is a lovely gesture to have bottles of water for them upon arrival. If there's any chance they'll be hungry, make sure there's a meal or snacks ready when they arrive. The first impression lasts, so arrange for a smooth and effortless arrival. If the rooms are cold, if they're shown to the wrong room or if they're left confused or hungry in the beginning, it will be harder for them to 'come down' and relax, which is such a big part of being on a yoga retreat. I have, in the past, had locally made eye bags waiting for everyone as a little gift, or left tea and personalised welcome notes on their beds. Depending on what time everyone arrives, you might dive right into a yoga class or a meal or just go to bed! Schedule accordingly, so their needs are met right off the bat and they feel neither rushed nor ignored.

Make sure you know where there is a local hospital, pharmacy and doctor. Know what the various excursions are, ideally from first-hand experience. Clarify any logistical issues early on with a welcome talk: where things are in the venue (the nearest bathroom to the yoga space for example), what other things are available to them (excursions, treatments) and what to expect from the yoga itself. You might choose to offer a half-day excursion at some point during the retreat to sightsee or go somewhere special as a group. In Morocco, we've gone hiking in the Atlas Mountains or gone shopping in Marrakech. In France, we went to a local market. In Egypt, we went snorkelling and hiked up Mount Sinai. In Sri Lanka, we went to the beach. In Thailand, we went to see a huge Buddha. This can vary from location and level of interest. There have also been retreats when the students were so tired they didn't want to go anywhere or do anything.

The retreat

Depending on the venue, length of time of the retreat, experience and needs of the students and what you actually teach, scheduling your yoga retreat is important. I have always asked students in advance of a retreat what they would like to work on during our time away, as well as what they're seeking from the whole experience. Sometimes the bulk of the guests report that they're exhausted and would like to relax; sometimes they report that they want to workshop certain poses or themes. It is important to honour whatever they request, with respect to the other students. It is tricky but vital to create a balance between strength and softness – perhaps stronger classes matched with meditation or restorative work. Rarely do students practise yoga as frequently at home as they will on the retreat, so you don't want to overwhelm or exhaust them.

One of the best parts of teaching a week-long (or longer) retreat is being able to work more consistently with the same group of students. You can establish language or patterns and build on them. You can take them on a journey into their practice and into themselves throughout the time. Usually, if there was a graph to demonstrate the energy levels of the group over a week, it would look something like the image below.

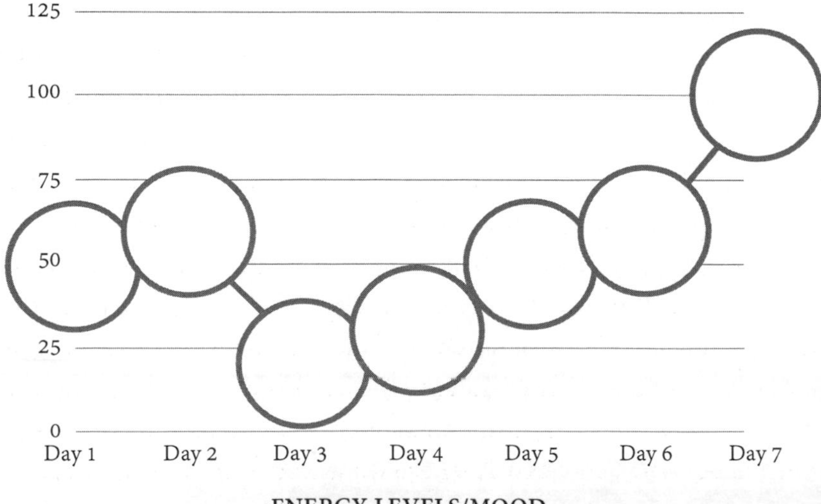

ENERGY LEVELS/MOOD

This is, of course, a generalisation and only applies if the retreat is one week in duration. But, for the most part, I have found it to ring true, no matter what age people are, what their professions are or how 'advanced' their practices are. People arrive on day one feeling pretty average: exhausted and stressed but used to this as 'the norm'. On day two they feel better, as they know they're on holiday and they are grateful and excited to be there. Then, on days three and four there's a slump, often when people feel more tired, grumpy and sore and experience odd or bad dreams. This is partly because they have really let go and are realising how run down they actually are/were, and partly because the yoga is working its magic and they're peeling back the tension and releasing the stress hormones. On days five and six the students feel better: seemingly overnight, they have more energy and a more positive outlook and are happier than before. It is hoped, then, that on day seven they will leave feeling much, much better than they did when they arrived.

I explain this, as it's important to consider in your sequencing of what you teach and when. It's important too to be aware of when you are 'holding space' for your students. Being compassionate during days two to four will allow the students to trust you enough to surrender their armour and truly open their hearts. Sometimes you can help this journey by teaching backbends on day three. But for the most part, the journey doesn't need provocation. In fact, I've found it more helpful to go with the graph and unlock them on days one to three with shoulders, hips and quieter more internal work to help them come down and then surf the wave of energy and openness during days five to seven with partner work, backbends or more open (perhaps more physical) work as well as deeper meditations and longer relaxations.

For the most part, I tend to find two classes a day works well. I teach two hours of dynamic practice in the morning and 1.5 hours of quiet practice (restorative, meditation and breath work) in the afternoon, but feel free to shift that or add more classes – whatever feels right to you and what you have to offer. All classes are tailored to all levels: I specialise in teaching open-level classes with options to suit levels 1, 2 and 3 practitioners. If you don't feel comfortable with that, you might schedule various classes to suit the various levels, like a level 1–2 class, a level 2–3 class and a class open to everyone. Keep in mind, though, how much you can comfortably teach without getting too tired.

Plan just enough that students feel taken care of, but also make sure they have downtime to themselves. Students who have come alone will cherish the time to nap, read and reflect. Students who have come as part of a couple or pair will enjoy spending time with their partners or friends. Be aware that there isn't really 'downtime' for you, necessarily. You will spend the time between classes sorting things for students, planning your next class, doing your own practice and getting to know the students better… My advice is to be available and easy to find all the time so it's easy for the students to ask for things or talk things through with you.

Carefully walk the line between professional and social – the students want access to you in between classes, so you might go on excursions with them or hang out by the pool with them, but you also want to maintain your professional image. It might go without saying, but don't get drunk during a retreat or show evidence of favouritism to some students over others. You are teaching not only during the set class times, but also by example. You are hosting as well as teaching. You are 'on call' 24/7 during the retreat period. On one retreat I had a student who needed an emergency root canal at 2am. Luckily, the hotel where we were staying was very helpful and responsible, so I was not alone in dealing with it.

The food during a retreat is important. Some retreats offer vegetarian menus that focus on being healthy and light; some offer meals that include everything, such as alcohol and desserts. I have taught both types of retreats and see value in both. Remember that you want the students to go home feeling great, so there is a lot to be said for strictly healthy meals. Yet the students are on holiday, so there is also a lot to be said for indulgent meals. It is vital to cater to any dietary requirements or allergies that the students have, without making them feel left out. If you're planning a retreat that will include meat, make sure the vegetarians get lovely options too and not just the side salads. Make sure there is enough protein on offer to keep energy levels up and there are regular snacks available so the students don't go hungry. Even if you're not focusing on a primarily health-conscious menu, it is always good to make sure there are balanced options that include a balance of protein, vegetables and carbohydrates. The students must stay hydrated, especially in hot climates. You might consider giving the students their own refillable water bottles to lessen the plastic waste. I have often given out water bottles at the beginning of the retreat that have the student's name on them, so they can refill them and there aren't lots of half-finished water bottles left lying around the yoga studio at the end of each class.

Some venues will include all food: three meals with perhaps two snacks. Some will only include bed and breakfast, and lunch and dinner will cost extra. Whatever it ends up being, make sure you are clear about it and that the students realise how much is included. For many years, I taught retreats in Egypt in which only breakfast was included, but lunch and dinner were very inexpensive so the students didn't mind at all, partly because I had warned them in advance. Lunch was ordered by the pool and we'd either eat dinner at the hotel or go into town. Buffets tend to work well, as there are various options and people can help themselves to what they want, as well as the portion size that works for them. I've often made snacks available first thing in the morning, along with teas (and, on some retreats, coffee) before class with the advice given to eat lightly to avoid being uncomfortable during yoga. Then we have brunch after morning class and options for lunch mid-afternoon and dinner after the afternoon/evening class. It's nice to facilitate everyone eating together but also to give space for those who want to eat alone or go on adventures with other guests. There is certainly benefit to having the first and last dinner (at the very minimum) all together as a group.

It's beautiful to witness the changes that occur during a retreat. Students let go more deeply than they can at home. Students find a softer, more open space within themselves. They make breakthroughs

– physically, mentally and emotionally. It is your job to support them through it and to create a space where they feel comfortable and safe enough to make these leaps.

Students often have emotional releases during retreats. If you feel grounded enough in yourself to do this, offer your ear to those who would like to talk. However, never give advice: you are not a counsellor or psychiatrist, just an open-minded, kind pair of ears. Help yourself energetically: you can feel burnt out if you take on their energy without cleansing it from yourself. I have, in the past, gone swimming in the sea after an emotional session with a student, visualising their sadness wash away from my own body. It's important to do your own practice – whatever that might be and however it might fit into the timetable of the retreat – so you too feel better at the end of the week. I used to find retreats particularly draining until I established techniques that worked for me to reground myself, as well as boundaries so as not to let students push me beyond what I'm able to handle.

If a student comes to you with any issue, listen to it thoroughly and see what you can do or perhaps how the venue can help you. If there's an issue with their room or the food, you can talk to the venue manager to resolve it (do, however, act as the middleman: don't ask the student go to the manager themselves as you are, after all, their host). If there's an issue such as the roommate you paired them with snores, see if you can move them so they share in a different room. If they become unwell, sort out a doctor's appointment for them either locally or even bring a doctor to the venue. It is common on international retreats for students to get funny tummies and need some local intestinal medicine in order to help them feel better. Act quickly to avoid it getting worse and to help the student feel taken care of.

Finally, be aware if a student is celebrating a birthday or important date during the retreat – an acknowledgement of it during the day can add a delightful personal touch. Once, at the closing of the morning class, I instructed the students to chant together. I said they all knew the words to that particular chant, and started singing happy birthday to one of the students. Everyone joined in and it was a lovely moment.

Heading home

I teach the final class as a 'bring-it-all-together' class: a little bit of everything we've done or worked on during the retreat. It's a great way for the students to chart their progress, remember elements you established earlier and 'seal in' the effects of their yoga. You might take a group photo to share with them upon return, but make sure you have permission from everyone in the photograph to share it with all the participants through email or post it on your social media or website if that's what you plan to do.

Consider how to make the journey home easier: do your students need packed snacks? Is the transport confirmed and clear to everyone? The students should settle their final bills before they check out – with you, the hotel, massage therapists, guides and so on. You don't want to chase them when you're home and they're back at work. Depending on whether you leave with them (in which case, you're still holding space until you part ways for a final time: I have students look to me to check the gate at the airport and I've even taught a seated stretch class at an airport when a flight was delayed) or after them (sometimes it's nice to stay an extra day to decompress for yourself), make sure the students are aware of what the next step is: will you email them? When can they work with you again? Will you set up any reunion lunches?

I have sold my DVDs and CDs at the end of a retreat, which for a while I resisted as I didn't want to seem opportunistic. However, I came around to the idea because I realised that students get in the habit of daily practice during retreats and they want to keep it going. It's a souvenir and a way to maintain their newly found sense of peace and joy when home. If that's not an option for you, make sure they know where to find you in the first week or so after they return home, so they don't lose momentum.

We did it!

When you've returned home, follow up with the students. Ask for feedback so you can better their experience next time. Consider offering discounts for booking on your next retreat (repeat customers are important in any business). Take stock for yourself on how you feel, what went well and what could have been better. Are you exhausted? Did your budget work out as you expected it to? Follow up with the venue, especially if you think you might go back. Give them feedback and thanks. Even if you don't think you might go back to that particular venue again, leave the relationship well enough that they welcome future yoga groups.

Conclusion

A retreat can be a magical and important experience to a yoga student: a time to break old patterns, make strides in their practice, 'go deeper', relax and rejuvenate. A retreat can be a fabulous experience for a yoga teacher, too: a time away from the everyday routine, space to work on elements of the practice that you don't have time to explore thoroughly in daily yoga classes. Plan your retreat in such a way that the experience is healing and restorative for all involved and it will be a new element to your teaching schedule that can bring you joy, satisfaction and profit in equal measures.

— 14 —

Setting Up a Yoga Studio

Paul Wong

Would you recommend starting a yoga studio or your own business? This question is often asked of me and I find it so difficult to answer because ultimately it comes down to every individual and their own dream, desire, drive and determination, and that is before even considering whether the business or studio 'idea' is feasible or likely to be a success. All I would say is if you truly believe you have what it takes to get over the line and you have a dream of running a yoga studio, then maybe it's time to get the wheels in motion, but do take time to do some serious soul-searching first. If opening a studio is your dream, then be ready for some hard work, unforeseen ups and downs and moments that truly test your yogic powers. And if you are ready to put the overall cause before yourself and your needs and energies, then you have what I believe it takes to open a studio that you will be proud of and one that you know you have put your heart and soul into. Then, on a day unknown, all that sweat, endeavour and outlaying of energy will start to come back to you in so many beautiful waves and ways as the community you have created starts to take shape.

We all have a dream and if opening a yoga studio is yours then you will have to approach this dream with a business mind to begin with because, for you to fulfil your dream, your idea has to work. And for a studio to work, the bottom line is that you will need enough students coming through the door to at least cover your outgoings. With this black-and-white bottom line in mind, before your ideas and dreams grow and evolve, do you feel that your initial studio plans, before anything is in place, will receive enough students through the door? This is a gut feeling that either says 'yes' or 'no'. If it's a 'yes', then what are you waiting for? If it's a 'maybe' then this is a good time to have a rethink – not of the whole dream but of certain aspects that turn the maybe into a 'yes'. If it's a 'no' then read through the below points and see if there are any major areas of adjustment, give your plans a rejig until you turn the 'no' into a 'yes' and then get the wheels in motion. This, of course, is by no means an exact science and there will be many things that surprise you in both good and bad ways along the way, no matter how much you plan. But if your initial gut feeling is strong then reach for that dream, push on and give it all you have.

There are many wonderful studios out there that are testament to the idea that opening a studio can work. Whether an intimate local studio or large-scale studio in the heart of a city, before starting on your journey of opening a studio, there are many practical points of consideration. Here are what I feel are some of the major points to be thinking on.

Area

Know your area and your potential student audience. Unless you really know the area in which you are considering opening a studio, you are going to be second guessing your audience and student base without some form of market research. This knowledge is essential when creating your studio feel and class styles, i.e. knowing what else is happening in the yoga scene in your preferred area. If the market is saturated within your dream area, it could be best to think of another area that has more of a calling for your studio.

If you know your area, and by that I mean knowing the main demographic, the overall energy, wellness awareness and what else is going on, you will be able to predict how your studio will 'go down' in the area you choose and be honest with yourself: is a yoga studio opening in the area likely to be well received? You don't want your dreams to cloud your judgement on this, so make sure the area feels right. We all know streets where we feel it would be beautiful to live, café's we wish were at the end of our road or the 'perfect area' for a yoga studio, but making this decision is not the time for daydreaming. Know your area and know, to the best of your ability, that there is a calling for what you wish to offer. If there is not a calling, you will have your work cut out in trying to build a community.

Like or live in your studio area. You will be spending a lot of time at and around the studio – within the first year or so your life will revolve around the studio – so I would recommend making your studio commute as easy as possible (possibly even relocating). Remember, every aspect of studio operation will fall on you (unless you have a studio manager on-board from the start): it is your responsibility seven days a week and at all hours of opening. Making sure all utilities are working, teachers are at the studio, toilets are stocked and cleaned: this daily list is possibly more extensive than you may first think. With this in mind, I think it is a good idea to live nearby, as running the studio can be hands on and your resources may be called on at any time.

These aspects may not be possible if you are already located and settled somewhere, but they are worth considering. Running a studio without a support network cannot be done remotely so you will have to be a physical presence at the studio to guarantee the smooth running.

Costs

'Whatever you think the costs will be, double it!' This is what was said to me at the start and this statement rang pretty much true. Once everything was finally in place and the time period established to get the wheels in motion, the actual financial outlay for setting up was nearing double the original estimate.

Even with the tightest and most well-thought-out budgets, there are many unforeseen outgoings of cash that soon start to add up, so make sure you factor this in. This is not to sound alarmist, but if you are starting to think about the financial side and if you are going to be purchasing or acquiring a lease and/or building your own studio, whatever your first estimate is, I would at least add another 50 percent and then I believe you will be nearer to what the final outlay for your project will be. This is unless, of course, you have taken on a similar project in the past, in which case make sure you use your previous experience to forecast and budget. One of the main things to consider is that the day you open the door doesn't indicate the day you start to gain a return on your investment. Building classes and a steady student following takes time and only in rare cases does this happen effortlessly and overnight. As a rough estimate, you could allow the following schedule from opening the doors: six months to break even; one year to stabilise and understand your studio better; two years to start to grow and establish. This timeline will vary greatly depending on the size and cost of the studio, whether you own or rent the property and all the other business outgoings, but from talking to others, this tends to be the rough trend.

If after working out a business and studio model you feel your idea is feasible financially, then there is no time like the present. It's up to you to make it a reality and this making of a reality will start with you having the finances in place.

There are numerous government initiatives for business start-ups and these are definitely worth exploring to get an idea of what potential help is out there. These schemes and initiatives change often so do your research and see what is available. There will probably be small business/entrepreneur hubs set up in your area. These can be a fantastic source of information and advice; I would strongly advise attending any group meetings within your target area and gaining as much knowledge and advice for business start-up that you can. Hearing other people's stories, struggles and high points can be a real eye-opener for getting a feel of the reality of starting your own business and they can provide invaluable lessons.

Financial circumstances vary for us all as well as the means of acquiring the necessary finances that will or will not be available to us. If a business bank loan is required, start doing your research and find out exactly what will be required from you. Start the groundwork and get advice on this now. I also know that crowdfunding has become a viable and successful means of raising the required finances and, again, if this is to be your means then start the enquiring now. Or maybe you have savings or family to help with this project; whatever your source and means, make sure you have the finances in place and remember the day the door opens is not the day you start to get a return: be prepared to tread water for a period.

The financing of a studio, like any business, is tough and needs to be approached and managed professionally. I guess the golden rules would be: do not underestimate the costs and don't overestimate your student numbers in the first year.

Property prices will vary between areas so it's a good idea to have a ballpark idea of what you get for your costs in a given area and whether the size of the space and predicted student numbers add up. This is somewhat of a guessing game or comes back to that gut feeling. If you feel your studio will have enough pull to finance and fill a 50-mat or multi-room studio, keep rolling with your dream. If you are aiming at a smaller local studio, the equation is exactly the same.

The day you open the door is the day your role changes from finding and setting up a studio to being the manager of the studio. You have to start to navigate the studio towards a stable point in the mould of how you wish it to be moving forward; be prepared for this change in role while carrying the financial weight of the studio.

Set up

You have found a space and gained the finances necessary for your project. Now for the studio set up. The main factors to consider are functionality, lighting, heating, noise, energy and upkeep. The set up of the studio will affect all these elements, and all these elements will affect your studio. When designing the layout, it is worth considering all these elements at every stage. Ultimately, you want to create a smoothly functioning studio with positive lighting, comfortable heating, low noise levels, a space that is easy to upkeep and a place where the overall energy is inspiring. All these points will vary on the size of your project and the space you have to work with. Very few studios are purpose-built so it's a case of making the best of your building framework. It's no good having the most beautiful studio space if it doesn't function correctly as a studio. Make sure the student and class experience is considered when designing every aspect of the layout.

When building the studio, like any building job, make sure you have professional people to help out on flooring, woodwork, plumbing, etc. and make sure you have the understanding to guide and direct the project correctly. It is more than likely that you will have to make changes along the way or once you have opened, so it's a good idea if you have built a relationship with some local trade professionals to help.

Once the main structure has been finalised, you have to make decisions on all the finer details. Mats, props, storage, music, plants, toilet facilities, refreshments…the list goes on. Remember: it is now down to you to make every last decision, so my advice would be to try to be good at making correct decisions but also be prepared to change and adjust as you go if something isn't working.

The set up is where you really start to see your dream coming together, so enjoy the process and put your love into it. Unless you have a large team on-board, the building and creating may take longer than you think, as small details and touches take time. You won't find everything under one roof or be able to rush the job. Enjoy the process and watch as your studio starts to take shape bit by bit.

Ethos

This is the thread that will connect all aspects of the business, including the website, studio and teachers. Take time to envisage not only your studio but also what you really want your studio to represent. Developing and creating your ethos will take time but it's sensible to always have a solid idea in mind when making decisions. Having a strong ethos running throughout will help with many aspects of the studio but mostly it will give you a voice with which to communicate. If you want to run a studio that is tied into the local area and you'd like to create a community around the studio, then all your communication, language, look, logo, etc. will have this ethos in mind. People need to know what you are about and, as far as possible, what to expect when going to the studio. Know your ethos and make sure everything ties back to this.

Experience

What is your yoga industry experience (and it is an industry – just as a studio has to be run as a business)? If it is limited, it may be a good idea to immerse yourself in the industry, especially if you are considering opening in a studio within a city. It's important to get an understanding of 'what's going on' but also for how things are done. Like any industry or venture, experience is vital. Although you learn a lot along the way, having a base knowledge and understanding are pretty vital for any business start-up, no matter how unique or good the idea is. If you don't have any experience or knowledge of the yoga industry or how to run a studio, it's time to do some groundwork. I've known people to 'karma yogi' at studios to gain a feel and experience of day-to-day studio life and what is involved in keeping a studio running smoothly and then go on to open their own studios.

If you have run your own yoga classes before, this will serve as great experience for moving into running a studio. You will understand that it is more than putting some mats on the floor, opening the door and magically students appearing to fill the room. The process takes time and hard work, with many ups and downs, but ultimately, when everything falls into place, it is richly rewarding. Building a following for a single class takes time and effort, and therefore building a following for a studio also takes time and effort. Apply all your past experience to your new project but understand there is a greater responsibility to carry. If you have rented a space and run your own class, you will have experienced the ups and downs. All week you are waiting, you've put in the work, spread the word as best as possible and you arrive, but no students follow. This then happens for the next two weeks and you start to doubt and to question, 'Is this worth the endeavour and financial outlay? Is there anyone out there?' Then, the following week, out of the blue the room is full of smiling students and your heart fills. You head home with a skip in your stride – all the effort seems more than worth it – this is your dream. And then the next week just one student shows and you question your teaching – what did you do wrong last week? This kind of rollercoaster of ups and downs is only magnified when running a studio and this is just the surface pressure. You will have to ride out this rollercoaster while carrying the financial strain of a studio and being the guiding light for all teachers and the studio as a whole. But on that day when you open the doors and see a room full of students, your heart and soul will fill and then you will know it was all worth it.

If you don't have experience, it may be advisable to get someone on-board who has the yoga experience. Some people who have nothing to do with the yoga industry open studios; they just enjoy yoga. This definitely can work, but I believe that at some point and for some decisions you need experience or to be prepared to learn quickly along the way. This often means making a few mistakes, but as long as you keep learning and moving forward, soon enough you will gain your own experience.

Teachers

Who will teach at your studio? Spending time with so many yoga teachers is one of the true joys of your role of running a studio. If you live in a city, there will more than likely be an abundance of teachers out there, perhaps available and willing to teach at your space. It's then up to you to choose which teachers you would love at your studio and to hope that the teachers will share that love of wanting to teach at your studio. Getting a timetable of teachers in place doesn't happen overnight and takes time and planning. Full-time yoga teachers tend to be self-employed and teach at many different studios. They have schedules that reflect this, so you cannot guarantee their availability. It takes times to build a timetable of teachers that reflects what your vision of the studio is. This ties in with your ethos and I believe helps with making decisions. You may have some teachers in mind who you connect with on a personal level and find inspiring, but you have to decide whether you feel the teacher will work at the studio or not; it's not your personal opinion that matters but what you feel is correct for the studio. This often doesn't come down to specific teaching but to the overall ethos and feel of the studio that you want to create. Once you have your teachers and timetable in place, just give them the studio support and platform to grow and teach. The actual choosing of teachers has to come down to you, so make sure you know what you want to try, and know which teachers are out there who could help you to create the studio and community that you want to grow.

Timeline

When you start out on this adventure, it is a good idea to have a timeline in mind, but remember your timeline is a guesstimate and things sometimes change or don't run as expected – be open to this. From the start, you will probably have set out a rough timeline along the lines of acquire the space, studio set-up, build the team, website, marketing and eventually open the doors. How long this all takes to get in place will vary greatly, but it's a good idea to know roughly how long you predict this setting up period taking. If you have the finances in place, this period can often be sped up by outsourcing and hiring skilled people to carry out certain aspects of the work for you. This will get you to the desired point quicker, but remember that unless you learn or understand the skills yourself you will always be calling on these people and outsourcing work. If you plan to keep everything 'in house' and learn as you go, expect your timeline to take longer and to have to put in a lot of physical and mental energy, the upside of which is that you will understand more aspects of your business. It is difficult to predict how long the first stages of building will take as there are many permutations that will affect this, but just ensure you have the finances and time available to see this period through. Acquiring any kind of property and building a facility will take patience and perseverance. You also have to be getting everything else prepared in the background, such as the studio website, timetable and marketing, and then you should aim for an open date and try your best to meet this.

Once the doors have opened, you will be working towards a timeline for student numbers and when you predict to start breaking even and making a living. This will tie in with your marketing and what methods you use to get the word out. If you have a very prominent studio front in a busy location, you may create a stir quite effortlessly, but if you are hidden away, you may have to shout a little louder. Just allow time for the studio to settle and grow, and don't expect full classes overnight. Achieving a loyal following and busy classes takes time and the best way to gain this is recommendations and word of mouth; this ties in with everything in your planning. As a rough timeframe, I would say you need six months to stabilise, find your feet and start to figure out what kind of following you will have and then you can start to grow and feel your way.

Marketing

Websites, Instagram, Facebook, flyering, emailing, PR campaigns and local collaborations… Marketing is a minefield and while some people love it, others have to hide from it. To some, it is a fine art; to others, a waste of time. But in some capacity, marketing will be essential for the survival and growth of your studio. Setting up a website is an integral part of your business and growing a mailing list is a great way of keeping your students on-board and informed. Know your website and try to get feedback from your students with regards to its usability and whether it represents the overall studio experience. The best method of marketing for you will depend on your area and student following. If you are in doubt or feel you need direction, using a marketing professional may be your best option to help direct you and the studio. In recent years, the yoga industry has flooded.

Instagram, with teachers and studios both using it as a platform to promote, inform and showcase. Whether you love it or hate it, Instagram appears to be the social platform that people are using today as an immediate means to advertise and promote. Instagram offers an immediate visual impact and also gives space for informing and promoting. As this is a worldwide platform, how effective it is for me is questionable, but as a visual and instantly informative platform it can work and it does give students an immediate, accessible source of up-to-date information. It is timely and instant, and once you get a handle on it, it's not too time consuming. But like all methods of marketing, you have to decide whether you wish to take this route and, if so, how you are going to approach it. As a studio we post a daily update of classes, teachers and any events. The satisfaction is knowing that we have done a little something extra to keep students informed, and whether we gain any extra students from this must be viewed as a bonus. There is a strong possibility that your teachers will have Instagram for their personal endeavours and this often links back to the studio in some way. It is like casting a very large net with no real specific catch in mind, but knowing the information and visual output are out there.

For more meaty and informative information, emailing and flyers can be a great way of getting your word out. We tend to send a monthly update that informs people of workshops and events for that coming month and any other news. And then, as mentioned above, we post a daily timetable update. You will get a lot of feedback about how regularly you should send emails, their effectiveness and so on, so again the decision is up to you. PR campaigns and local collaborations are also often used as a means of promoting a studio, its teachers and other events. Working with other businesses such as cafés within your area can be a great way to boost awareness and help form local bonds within the community. Get help with or make a choice about what marketing tools you wish to use and try to learn what works best for you and the studio. Trying out all methods of marketing and then analysing what was most effective with regards to time, cost and feedback could be best at the start to establish which method suits or lends itself to your studio. What works for some won't work for others, but unless you are the only studio within the area and have a instant following of dedicated and loyal students, you will have to partake in some form of marketing. Choose a direction and follow it through or get the advice of a professional.

Setbacks

Within the first year of operating (unless you have run a studio before), all is going to be new and involve some kind of learning. Do what you can to keep things running as smoothly as you can, but be flexible in your dealing with setbacks – they happen. What these setbacks will be is hard to say, but in the first year it is advisable to be on your toes and at least have systems and fall-back ideas in place to cope with issues that arise. These may be related to the building you occupy, such as damp, flooding, utility issues or plumbing problems, or they may be related to the day-to-day running of the studio, such as teachers leaving, injuries, last-minute cancellations, lost keys…the list goes on. Just remember to do what you can to keep the studio running smoothly and when problems arise, do what you can to deal with them and then get back to the day-to-day running. The more experience you gain, the better you adapt and react to these issues and the more systems you will have in place to resolve and pre-empt.

Highlights

You open the doors on a sunny day, classes are busy with smiling faces, you have uplifting chats with students and teachers, you realise that the studio is part of the community and the space has become a sanctuary for you and the students. Someday it will just hit you, and you add to the glow and energy of the place, you have manifested your dream, you are in tune with your destiny and you feel the difference you have made to the community. Does it get much better than that?

But why a yoga studio? This is a question you will have to ask yourself seriously before embarking on this adventure. Once you know the reasons for opening your studio, you have the main driving force behind your studio. Once you have asked yourself this question, many different reasons are going to arise. To make a living, to be in and around 'yoga' on a full-time basis, to build a community, to make a change for the good within people's lives, to create a brand, to create a sacred space – whatever the motivation is, there has to be a strong reason and passion behind that. I believe you have to have a strong passion and reason for opening a studio beyond the initial idea and dream, because during the tough times, this is what you can pull your strength from. Knowing that the reason you are at the studio seven days a week is that you have a burning desire to create a community and space for people means that you want to be there seven days a week. Knowing that you want to be in and around all things yoga means you will be happy to fully commit to it seven days a week and live and breathe the studio and all things yoga, as this has been your burning life passion. Whatever the reason, know deep down why you want to open a studio, as you won't really be able to feel a sense of fulfilment unless this is known. If you know the reason you want to open a studio is to create a 'yoga brand', you won't feel satisfaction until the day that you feel you have created this brand in the way you dreamed it to be.

Know why you want to open a studio, be true and honest with yourself and then drive towards that with all you have. I believe this is essential. Any business start-up, no matter what business, takes full commitment. Unless this venture is a hobby or a sideline and you have the finances, resources and energy to run it from a distance with minimum participation, running a studio is more than a full-time job and takes complete attention and nurturing. Therefore, knowing your reason for opening a studio will give you the drive when you wake up in the morning.

It is hoped the studio will grow and change as time passes, and with this your roles will change and your energy outlay will start to move with the studio. For me, the amount of admin, background work and email communication was greatly underestimated, especially as classes got busier and more teachers become involved. So, as your role and maybe your hours of teaching (if you are a teacher) change or your hours at the studio start to reduce, knowing your initial reason for opening may be a place of comfort as you wade through hours of admin. Remembering that whatever your role in this is or becomes, your reason for opening remains the same, and it is hoped your love and passion will remain intact.

Search deep and know the reason why you want to do this, be honest with yourself and then all that is left to do is get the ball rolling. Opening a studio is a challenging experience with many points of learning along the way, but the moments of magic and wonder that come back in return make the rollercoaster a ride worth taking. Who knows how many lives the studio will positively influence and inspire?

—— 15 ——

Case Studies

Lessons Learned from New and Established Teachers

Sian O'Neill

This chapter includes a few case studies with teachers at different stages in their yoga teaching careers. I have personally found it helpful to learn from other teachers, including their tips from experience and words of advice. It can be reassuring just to know that others are experiencing the same issues or challenges as you. I hope that you take something away from the case studies below that you find useful in your own yoga teaching.

Vanessa Hartley, two years qualified

From a jazz dance background, Vanessa was introduced to yoga at Pineapple Studios, practising power yoga and enjoying its effects. Vanessa has always been spiritual, meditating from the age of 21 and learning how to quieten the mind through the breath in her mid-20s.

Vanessa also mentions that she ran a pub in the centre of London, increasing the pub's profits substantially while practising yoga on breaks. Vanessa clearly also has a commercial head. After a period of time, her 'soul said change' and she realised she needed to move on. She trained with Tarik Dervish, drawn by the five days at the Mandala Ashram, which she loved, and Tarik's authentic approach. When asked which aspects of the course she particularly liked, she mentions anatomy as offering another layer to her knowledge and teaching. She enjoyed the thorough British Wheel of Yoga training and the depth of the course. There were 16 students on her course, which she thought was a good number and she felt the group became a lovely community. Vanessa started teaching while on the course and graduated two years ago.

Her first class teaching ended up being cancelled and Vanessa experienced a real reluctance to put a CV together. Something was holding Vanessa back and, as she also practises energy work, she applied it to herself to let go of what she needed to leave behind.

She now teaches ten classes a week, including some private classes and her energy work alongside. She is not sure whether she wants to take on additional classes. I sense that, with her vibrant energy, Vanessa could possibly take on too much, with which she agrees. She has considered the optimal number of classes for her and, for example, made the decision not to cross London for different classes and thereby spend most of her time on transport.

When asked what yoga means to her, Vanessa replies that it has become her life: 'I am yoga.' She enjoys the sense of connection in a class – offering students what they need with fun and lightness. In fact, the concept of connection recurs throughout our conversation: she enjoys connecting people to their bodies, breath and other people.

To support herself and her practice, Vanessa attends three to four classes a week, trying out different teachers (she is not a fan of yoga teacher gurus), and has a strong home practice. She also finds support from other yoga teachers. She enjoys sitting still, not necessarily meditating but just 'being'. As an energy worker, she is aware of the impact of working with other people's energies and finds just sitting still, sometimes for an hour at a time, beneficial. She also finds teaching grounding for herself.

When asked what advice Vanessa would give to new teachers, she says to 'trust yourself' and 'don't feel pressure'.

Alison Leighton, five years qualified

Alison's background was previously in human resources and law in London, and she led a somewhat hectic lifestyle. Yoga was recommended as a way to slow down and, although she didn't enjoy her first class, Alison returned a couple of years later and became interested very quickly, increasing both her strength and flexibility in a short space of time. Her practice at that stage was a mixture of slow and strong (Iyengar and Hatha) yoga but is now more anchored in a Vinyasa Flow practice.

Inspired to deepen her knowledge and learn more, Alison signed up for the Triyoga teacher training in 2010–2012. She advises those considering training to research carefully the different courses on offer. She loved her course and particularly liked the strong philosophy component offered by Triyoga. She has used this solid foundation in philosophy to weave into her own classes. When asked if she would have appreciated more coverage on any particular aspects, she mentions the business of running your yoga career plus adjusting, which could perhaps have been covered in more depth.

Alison started teaching while on the course in 2010 and stresses the importance of planning classes around a theme, which could be anatomical or, for example, philosophical (such as around boundaries or the chakras). She is currently training to be a transpersonal psychotherapist and finds that a source of inspiration when planning themes for classes.

Post-qualification, Alison is an active learner, attending workshops, British Wheel of Yoga online study courses and the year-long Urban Priestess course with Sianna Sherman. She also uses Yoga International and attends classes, two of her regular teachers being contributors Liz Lark and Tanja Mickwitz.

When asked what being a yoga teacher means to her, Alison replies that it is a way of life and that she is doing something that feels right. Alison gains much satisfaction from sharing the practice of yoga with her clients and enjoys teaching people of all levels. Interestingly, Alison has written a yoga teaching manifesto that sets out her vision for her yoga teaching career and the steps to get there and includes where she would like to be in the next few years, echoing the importance of intention referred to by other contributors within this book.

Her advice for yoga teachers once qualified is to consider what type of yoga they want to teach: what is your offering and what differentiates you? She also recommends paying attention to accounting and keeping track of your income and expenses when teaching yoga is your main job. When Alison started teaching, she accepted all teaching opportunities in order to get herself established and suggests other teachers might do the same, as there are peaks and troughs in teaching. Alison initially covered classes and now has her own permanent classes as well as teaching one-on-one. She mentions that the best advice she was given was to have her own, regular practice and a clear intention of where she would like to take her business: 'have a vision'.

To relax, Alison practises yoga and takes a class once a week. She also enjoys chanting, singing along to mantras (such as Deva Premal), Thai massage, reading novels and gardening. It is clear that Alison is very organised and pays attention to intelligent scheduling, for example, keeping the weekend clear and condensing classes from Monday to Thursday, leaving Friday open for her charity work (she works with a child bereavement charity) or other activities.

A day in the life of Alison Leighton

5.40am	The early morning alarm goes off and I get ready to meet a private client who lives close by.
6–7am	I spend an hour with my client. We discuss what she would like from the practice before we start to move.
7.15–9am	Return home, eat breakfast and catch up on the day's news.
9am	Travel to Canary Wharf where I teach a group class. As I'm often travelling on public transport, I will usually have my head in a novel.
10.15–11am	Teach a Vinyasa Flow yoga class to the employees of a large bank.

11.15am	Return home, grabbing some groceries en route, and eat a light lunch.
12.45–2pm	Take a local yoga class with Tanja Mickwitz, one of my favourite teachers.
2.30pm–4pm	Back at home, I'll spend some time doing any of the following: Planning classes: I develop a theme each week that I structure classes around. Some weeks the theme might need more research than other weeks. I vary the theme and sequencing slightly depending on the class level and length of the class. Keep my accounts up to date: it has to be done. This involves logging all classes I teach, issuing invoices, checking invoices have been paid and recording all business expenses. I'm always on the look out for new, interesting music to play in my classes, so I might spend time listening to new releases online. • Marketing: I spend time promoting my teaching and growing my client base. • I also spend time keeping up to date by reading journals. • I am training to be a psychotherapist so I spend time studying. Separately, I provide bereavement counselling services to children on behalf of a local charity as part of my training.
4–5.15pm	Relaxing and/or catching up on all things domestic.
5.15pm	Travel to Covent Garden to cover a yoga class.
6–7pm	Teach a Vinyasa Flow yoga class.
7.30pm	Return home, prepare dinner with my husband and then relax.
10pm	Bedtime.

Alison Purchase, over 12 years qualified

Alison started practising yoga whilst at university in Canada when she was around 18, dipping in and out of different classes.

At around 21, Alison moved to England and, not knowing anyone, joined a gym and started going to yoga classes regularly. It was there that she met Terry Reader, who became something of a mentor at that stage. He invited her to join a small private class in the *Sivananda* style of around five students, which Alison loved, finding them calming and giving her an opportunity to deepen her practice.

On Terry's advice, Alison explored teacher training options and applied for one of the very first intakes of teacher training at The Life Centre. Although challenging at first, she found the course thorough and in-depth, setting her up properly for teaching yoga. She started teaching while on the course, assisting Mark Ansari, a mentor on the course, covering some of Terry's classes at a gym in north London and teaching at Dance Attic, where she taught for many years and which she loved. She also rented a room at the North London Buddhist Centre in Islington, where she still teaches two yoga classes a week. In retrospect, she wouldn't have chosen to rent a room, as only a couple of classes with a small number of students or no students is enough to wipe out any profits. She was then invited to join the regular roster of teachers, so moving on to the payroll. One of Alison's tips for new teachers is to learn about registering as self-employed, which was covered in her teaching training.

At one point, Alison was teaching five classes per week on top of a full-time job. When asked how she managed to juggle the two, Alison replies that she actually found it easier to teach this many classes while working full-time and in the working mode. There was just one class later in the evening that she found more challenging as it meant she arrived home late. She only started to cut down the number of classes when she became pregnant with her little boy. Her advice to teachers considering taking on new classes while working full-time is not to take on too many and to be realistic if you are not going to reduce the number of hours in the day job. She also advises being careful about weekend classes if working full-time.

Alison's motivation to teach is that she loves yoga and loved learning about the philosophy and history of yoga, so it also stems from an academic interest. She loves sharing knowledge, teaching (at one point, Alison considered becoming a school teacher) and feeling the energy of the students.

Alison also advises newer teachers to take on covers and thinks this is important while training. Alison herself took on many covers for Terry earlier on in her career and benefited from the challenge of teaching a class where you don't know anyone and where people might even be resistant to you as a cover teacher.

Alison doesn't have a written plan for classes but she does follow a broad framework, which she then fills in from her repertoire of poses. She starts off with a warm up, moving on to Sun Salutations (which she varies creatively), standing postures, balances, hip openers, backbends or moving more deeply into hip openers and then twists and forward bends. She enjoys the flexibility of being able to slot in different poses within a broad framework and believes that the lack of a rigid class plan enables her to adapt classes according to who is in the class. She quite often structures classes towards a peak pose.

Being a yoga teacher to Alison means sharing yourself and, although that can be draining, she also takes back energy from the class. On that note, Alison strongly believes that a yoga teacher holds the energy of the class and should, for example, be the first to open the door at the end of a class – that you as a yoga teacher 'hold' the room. She also believes a yoga teacher needs to stick to the allotted time for the class and that to run over implies that your time is more important than that of the students. She also believes it is important to offer modifications and alternatives for poses – that a yoga teacher should not be a dictator and needs to have an element of understanding and softness.

To relax, Alison loves baths and the outdoors. Although a city girl, Alison loves the country and being by water. She also reads a lot.

In terms of future plans, Alison would like to teach children (having already completed a training to teach children). She would also like to learn to teach pregnancy yoga and to hold a retreat. She believes that going on further trainings reinvigorates you as a teacher.

Alison's top 10 tips for new yoga teachers

- **Keep your class plan flexible.** Plan the general structure of a class rather than each pose. That way you can adapt the class based on the students' needs and you won't feel stressed if you forget what pose you had planned next.
- **Take an interest in your students.** If you arrive early and stay late, you have the opportunity to chat with your students and find out more about them. Students often have questions or are looking for advice to develop their practice.
- **Be creative.** Unless you teach Ashtanga, don't do the same sequence of poses every week. I like to be creative with Sun Salutations and while I have a particular style and structure to my class, I do different poses every week to keep things fresh.
- **Keep to time.** Running over in a class sends the message that your time is more important than the students'.
- **Give modifications.** All your students will be at different levels and places in their lives. There is no point in pushing someone to do something they aren't ready to do. Providing modifications that are easier and more challenging than the base pose means students can go at their own pace. This is especially important in drop-in or general classes where you'll get a wide range of students with different needs and abilities.
- **Stay calm.** Students expect a relaxed and confident teacher, so keep your composure even if you've had a terrible day or you draw a blank. If you need time to think about what pose to go

to next, put the class into Down Dog or Child Pose while you think about it.

- **Try not to get overly concerned with students' facial expressions.** When people concentrate, they can look bored, confused or even angry. Chat to your students after the class to find out how they got on.
- **Don't overdo the number of classes you commit to.** Be realistic on what you can balance with your personal life and any other work you're doing, especially if you work full-time. When you teach you're sharing your energy; taking on too many classes can cause burnout. If you're feeling stressed or overwhelmed, this will come across in your teaching.
- **Don't speak for the sake of speaking.** You don't need to speak the entire time; choose your words mindfully and give your class the space to reflect on their practice and their breathing by allowing some quiet pauses throughout your class.
- **Maintain the energy of the room.** As the teacher, you hold the energy of a room. Be the first person to open the door at the end of the class to release the energy and never leave the class during the relaxation.

About the Authors

Katy Appleton

katy@appleyoga.com

Katy Appleton, Founder and Director of appleyoga, brings to yoga more than 25 years of expertise in movement through ballet, Pilates, body tuning, breath and energy work. She is an internationally recognised teacher of Vinyasa Flow and is known for bringing the true essence of yoga alive in a student's body-mind in creative, dynamic and life-transforming ways. Her teaching is biomechanically savvy whilst fun and playful, invoking a deeper embodied sense of self within a practice.

Her integrated teaching style involves an eclectic mix of Dynamic Vinyasa, Bhakti yoga, (the heart essence path), structured alignment, philosophy, mantra, Sufi poetry and wicked musical vibes. She draws on her experiences to form her own style of yoga, known worldwide as appleyoga. Katy is also the creator of the appleyoga school, running life-transforming teacher trainings, apple adventure worldwide retreats and online courses. She has published several yoga books and award-winning DVDs for home practice. For more information about Katy and appleyoga visit www.appleyoga.com.

Antonia Boyle

alphawavesnlp@aol.com

Antonia Boyle is a Master Practitioner Neuro Linguistic Programming (NLP) and qualified NLP Health Specialist. She is director of Training of Alpha Waves International PDS. She uses NLP in her Outcome

Focused Coaching Brief Therapy Practice and training programmes. She works as a trainer, coach and therapist with a wide range of people. For the last 20+ years, a large part of her work has been working one to one with clients at the Westerham NLP Practice in Kent. Her other areas of expertise are yoga, meditation and relaxation. She trained yoga teachers for more than 20 years for the British Wheel of Yoga. Her two-day NLP for Yoga Teachers course is recognised by the British Wheel of Yoga as part of their continuing education programme for yoga tutors. She has produced a CD four-part relaxation mini course, which combines NLP with relaxation: www.alphawavesnlp.co.uk/untangle-your-mind-relax-your-body.html. Visit her website for further information on courses: www.alphawavesnlp.co.uk.

Graham Burns

grahamyoga@hotmail.com

Graham Burns has taught yoga professionally since 2001, principally at The Life Centre and Triyoga in London. Graham teaches yoga history, philosophy, Sanskrit and meditation on the Yogacampus Yoga Teacher Training Diploma courses in London, Manchester and Yorkshire, and also serves as a board member for the Manchester and Yorkshire courses, as well as leading workshops and trainings in the UK and abroad. His main yoga teaching influences over the years have been Richard Freeman, Rod Stryker and Simon Low.

As well as a law degree from a previous life, Graham has an MA (with Distinction) in Indian Religions from SOAS, University of London, where he has also lectured on the MA course in Traditions of Yoga and Meditation and teaches undergraduate Hinduism. He is currently completing his PhD at SOAS on the development of teachings on ultimate reality in the *Vedic Upaniṣads*.

Melanie Cooper

xmelaniexx@yahoo.co.uk

Melanie has been teaching yoga for 20 years. She is passionate about making yoga safe and right for everyone individually. She mainly divides her time between England and Goa, practising and teaching yoga and sometimes dancing on the beach. For many years she was running the morning Mysore programme at The Life Centre, one of London's most prestigious yoga centres. She now lives in Bristol and runs regular classes, workshops, teacher trainings and retreats in UK, Europe and India and is the author of *Teaching Yoga Adjusting Asana*.

Tarik Dervish

tarik@yogawell.co.uk

Tarik Dervish holds an honours degree in *Āyurveda* and has had 15 years of clinical experience in the field. He is also a Teacher Trainer, Verifier and Modules Officer for the British Wheel of Yoga, the largest yoga organisation in the UK.

He has a passion for educating the yoga community in the basic principles of *Āyurveda* and has been running courses and workshops in *Āyurveda* for Yoga practitioners since 2001. He also runs Yoga Foundation and Teacher Training courses in London and Brighton.

He has a special interest in techniques that work with the 'energy body' and his teaching is inspired by ancient tantric techniques as well as a variety of other healing modalities.

He is a regular contributor to *Spectrum* magazine and is also involved in a health charity called the Helios Foundation that works with less advantaged people living with chronic health conditions.

He lives in Brighton and runs workshops all over the country. For more information about his work, visit www.yogawell.co.uk.

Vanessa Hartley

vanessa@yogaisforlife.com

Having trained as a dancer when she first started practising yoga, Vanessa approached it with much the same mentality. All from ego! It reflected her lifestyle of bouncing around from job to job, busy, busy, busy.

After having her son, Vanessa knew her life was changing direction and yoga was beginning to play a major part in that change. Trusting the signs and synchronicity, she was lucky enough to find Tara Fraser, who started her on the path of becoming a yoga teacher, expanding her knowledge in yoga philosophy with guidance to deepen her practice. Vanessa met Tarik Dervish who, being so grounded and honest with his teachings, really gave her the confidence to be the teacher she is today. She is forever grateful.

Although life can still be busy, with her red Dr Martens on her feet and yoga mat over her shoulder, she could not be happier!

Lisa Kaley-Isley

lisa@lifetreeyoga.co.uk

Lisa Kaley-Isley is a practising yoga teacher, yoga therapist and yoga therapy educator in London. Lisa is on the Board of Directors for the Yogacampus Yoga Therapy Diploma course. She teaches and supervises students on the course and is Director of the Yoga Therapy Clinic in Islington. Lisa is a long-term student of Yogarupa Rod Stryker and Pandit Rajmani Tigunait in the Para Yoga and Himalayan Institute traditions. She received yoga therapy training in the American Viniyoga tradition with Gary Kraftsow. Lisa earned her PhD in Clinical Psychology in the US in 1992. From 1998 until her move to the UK in 2009, Lisa served in various roles at The Children's Hospital, Colorado including Director of Psychology Training, Chief of Psychology and founding Clinical

Director of the Pediatric Integrative Medicine Program. She conducted research into the effectiveness of yoga for reducing symptoms of anxiety, depression and somatisation in adolescents diagnosed with medical and mental health disorders exacerbated by stress. She presented her findings at conferences across the US and has published articles on yoga for adolescents.

Mimi Kuo-Deemer

mimi@mkdeemer.com

Mimi has been a student of yoga since 1995 and an avid lover of dance since 1978, when her mother put her in ballet school for walking with turned-in toes. Her two main teachers in the yoga world are Erich Schiffmann and Donna Farhi. Her qigong practice, inspired by her own curiosity and love for Daoism and the Chinese Five Elements, emerged as a complementary and distinct practice alongside her love of yoga and meditation.

Originally from Tucson, Arizona, Mimi spent 13 years living in China, where she co-founded and co-directed Yoga Yard, Beijing's first and leading yoga centre. She now lives in London, where she is a senior teacher and teacher-training faculty member at Triyoga. She contributes to movementformodernlife.com, is the author of the DVD *Vinyasa Yoga: A Steady, Mindful Practice* and has a Masters with distinction in Traditions of Yoga and Meditation from SOAS, University of London. www.mkdeemer.com

Liz Lark

astangayogalark@hotmail.com

Liz Lark is a yoga artist, enriched with an arts background (MA, BA degrees in Ceramic Sculpture and Performing Arts). She has been teaching yoga since 1995, after a strong foundation in Hatha yoga

(British Wheel of Yoga teacher training) and Ashtanga Vinyasa (Derek Ireland in Crete and Goa). A creative, mindful approach to body-mind nourishment underlies her teaching, inspired with visual imagery and body poetics to prompt philosophy. Sequencing forms a rich thread like a coloured river through her teaching, pausing for contemplation, cultivating fluid strength within safe Vinyasa Kramas. Liz teaches workshops, retreats and has written many books, with a DVD and online teaching (M4ML, Yoopod). See her website to join a retreat: Liz Lark Yoga Art at www.lizlark.com.

Lizzie Lasater

jai@lizzielasater.com

Raised in San Francisco and trained as a designer, Lizzie Lasater M.Arch, RYT, teaches restorative yoga internationally and online.

She sometimes jokes that yoga 'runs in the family' because her mom, Judith Hanson Lasater, co-founded *Yoga Journal Magazine* and has been teaching since 1971.

Lizzie posts daily on Instagram about the pleasure of deceleration. She lives in the Alps with her Austrian husband. www.lizzielasater.com

Alison Leighton

yogaalison@yahoo.com

Alison's yoga journey began in 2006 when she fell in love with the practice of linking movement with breath. Since then, yoga has become an integral part of her life.

Alison trained at Triyoga and is certified by the British Wheel of Yoga. Alison has been teaching in central London since 2010. Her earlier careers were in law and human resources. Alison teaches a heart-felt, creative Vinyasa Flow practice inspired by a range of yoga traditions.

In addition to teaching yoga, Alison is currently training to become a transpersonal psychotherapist.

Further details, including Alison's current schedule, can be found at www.yogaalison.co.uk.

Andrew McGonigle

mcgonigleandrew@hotmail.com

After originally training to become a doctor, Andrew McGonigle moved away from Western medicine to pursue a career as a yoga teacher, massage therapist and anatomy teacher.

Based in both London and Los Angeles, Andrew has been practising yoga and meditation for 15 years and teaching strong, grounding, alignment-based yoga since 2009.

Andrew combines all of his skills to teach anatomy and physiology on yoga teacher training courses across the world.

He contributes monthly to *Om Yoga & Lifestyle Magazine* with his 360° Yoga anatomy feature and has released a series of anatomy-applied-to-yoga apps.

His teachers include Hamish Henry, Paul Dallaghan, Eileen Gauthier, Kristin Campbell, Anna Ashby and Sally Kempton.

For more information please visit: www.doctoryogi.co.uk.

Tanja Mickwitz

tanjamickwitz@gmail.com

Known for her authentic voice and for speaking from the heart, Tanja weaves yogic principles and life understanding into a journey of creative flow and intelligently progressed *āsana*. Her Soulful Vinyasa classes serve as an inspiration and support for life, with *āsana* as the playground and metaphor. Tanja creates a nurturing space for exploration of the internal landscape and inner growth whilst challenging the physical edge with a safely led dynamic practice. Tanja is also an engaging storyteller and teaches regular Mythical Flow classes where she weaves the Indian deities, their stories and symbolism into the practice.

Tanja is based in London where she is one of the senior teachers at The Life Centre in addition to being a teacher and mentor for Yogacampus Teacher Training. She is registered SYT (Senior Yoga Teacher) with Yoga Alliance UK and E-RYT 200 and RYT 500 with Yoga Alliance US. *www.tanjamickwitzyoga.com*

Natasha Moutran

natasha@natashamoutran.com

Natasha Moutran is the Co-Founder of The Retreat Collection and an international yoga and meditation teacher. Natasha started her journey as a teacher out of the love and joy of her yoga practice and her wish to share this with London and around the world. She has been teaching for over six years, offering retreats and classes both in London and across the globe, sharing her love of yoga and meditation wherever she goes.

Having trained with appleyoga, Natasha has gone on to study with a number of inspiring teachers, gaining further insight into this realm in order to offer more through her teachings and is currently completing her 1000 hours in Yoga Medicine. Natasha continues to work with appleyoga and is an appleyoga teacher and mentor on the appleyoga Teacher Trainings.

Natasha has since gone on to become the Co-Founder and Director of The Retreat Collection, a luxury boutique retreat company offering transformational and beautiful retreats around the world.

Sian O'Neill

sianoneill@yahoo.co.uk

Believing in the transformational power of yoga, Sian has been practising yoga for around 14 years. She completed the British Wheel of Yoga accredited teacher training diploma at Yogacampus and also the British Wheel of Yoga Ayurvedic Yoga Therapy module with Tarik Dervish and the Scaravelli Immersion course with Catherine Annis.

She attends regular workshops and has been fortunate to learn from eminent practitioners, including the wise and experienced tutors at Yogacampus and from intensives/workshops with leading practitioners from around the world.

Sian teaches a flowing Hatha yoga class incorporating alignment, a mindful flow and breath awareness, aiming to help students on their own path of yoga. She is also a regular contributor of yoga-related articles including to *Spectrum* magazine, the official magazine of the British Wheel of Yoga.

Further details can be found at www.yogawithsian.co.uk.

Alison Purchase

alipurchase77@gmail.com

Alison Purchase is a Canadian-born yoga teacher who trained in the first intake of The Life Centre/ Yogacampus teacher training and qualified as a yoga teacher in 2005. She has been practising yoga for 21 years and teaching for 13 years in centres around London, including the Dance Attic, Camden Physio Centre, St Pancras Physio Centre and the North London Buddhist Centre where she currently teaches two classes a week. She also holds qualifications in nutrition and teaching yoga to children. Alison draws on elements from Ashtanga, Sivananda, Hatha and Vinyasa yoga to create her class plan. Her style of teaching combines dynamic flow with creative sequencing to bring balance and flexibility to the body and mind.

Kate Walker

katewalkeryoga@gmail.com

Having grown up in New York and Los Angeles, Kate Walker started studying yoga in 1998. She was the weakest, most inflexible person in the yoga room, but persevered, as the quiet and calm internal state was unlike anything she had ever known. Having now taken part in numerous teacher trainings, she credits Max Strom, Edward Clark, Seane Corn, Annie Carpenter, Judith Lasater and Rodney Yee as her main influences.

Kate specialises in teaching all level classes with a balance of mindful, strong, breath and alignment-based Vinyasa Flow with restorative yoga and relaxation. She teaches retreats worldwide. She is one of the most popular teachers at Europe's largest yoga venue, Triyoga in London, where she teaches regular classes and workshops. She has released two DVDs, one an all levels Vinyasa yoga DVD, and one a restorative yoga and relaxation DVD, both available through her website: katewalkeryoga.com.

Paul Wong

hello@mudrayogalondon.com

Paul is Owner and Teacher at Mudra Yoga London based in Stoke Newington in North/East London. He started out renting and running yoga classes from various community spaces around London with his partner and fellow yoga teacher Emily-Clare Hill before they decided to open their own studio. These formative years and the experience of running community-based classes provided the ethos and ideas behind Mudra to provide a friendly and accessible community-orientated yoga studio with expert, passionate teachers. Ever present at the studio, Paul is the heartbeat of Mudra and takes great pride in providing an open space for students to feel welcome and inspired when they come to practise. Paul's drive for community wellbeing and positivity shines through every class and is at the core of everything at the studio.

Index

Please note that page references to End Notes will be followed by the letter 'n' and number of the Note.